100.89

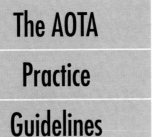

The AOTA
Practice
Guidelines
Series

Occupational Therapy
Practice Guidelines *for*

Driving and Community Mobility for Older Adults

Wendy B. Stav, PhD, OTR/L, SCDCM
Assistant Professor
Department of Occupational Therapy and Occupational Science
Towson University
Towson, Maryland

Linda A. Hunt, PhD, OTR/L
Associate Professor
School of Occupational Therapy
Pacific University
Forest Grove, Oregon

Marian Arbesman, PhD, OTR/L
Clinical Assistant Professor
Department of Rehabilitation Science
School of Public Health & Health Professions
University at Buffalo
Buffalo, New York
Consultant
AOTA Evidence-Based Practice Project

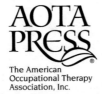
AOTA
PRESS
The American
Occupational Therapy
Association, Inc.

Vision Statement

AOTA advances occupational therapy as the pre-eminent profession in promoting the health, productivity, and quality of life of individuals and society through the therapeutic application of occupation.

Mission Statement

The American Occupational Therapy Association advances the quality, availability, use, and support of occupational therapy through standard-setting, advocacy, education, and research on behalf of its members and the public.

AOTA Staff

Frederick P. Somers, Executive Director
Christopher M. Bluhm, Chief Operating Officer
Audrey Rothstein, Director, Marketing and Communications

Maureen Peterson, MS, OT/L, FAOTA, Chief Professional Affairs Officer
Deborah Lieberman, MHSA, OTR/L, FAOTA, Program Director, Evidence-Based Practice, Practice Department
V. Judith Thomas, MGA, Senior Policy Manager

Chris Davis, Managing Editor, AOTA Press
Rick Ludwick, Project Manager
Timothy Sniffin, Production Editor II
Carrie Mercadante, Editorial Assistant

Robert A. Sacheli, Manager, Creative Services
Sarah E. Ely, Book Production Coordinator

Marge Wasson, Marketing Manager
Stephanie Heischman, Marketing Specialist
John Prudente, Marketing Specialist

The American Occupational Therapy Association, Inc.
4720 Montgomery Lane
Bethesda, MD 20814
Phone: 301-652-AOTA (2682)
TDD: 800-377-8555
Fax: 301-652-7711
www.aota.org

To order: 1-877-404-AOTA (2682)

Disclaimers

This publication is designed to provide accurate and authoritative information in regard to the subject matter covered. It is sold or distributed with the understanding that the publisher is not engaged in rendering legal, accounting, or other professional service. If legal advice or other expert assistance is required, the services of a competent professional person should be sought.
—*From the Declaration of Principles jointly adopted by the American Bar Association and a Committee of Publishers and Associations*

It is the objective of the American Occupational Therapy Association to be a forum for free expression and interchange of ideas. The opinions expressed by the contributors to this work are their own and not necessarily those of the American Occupational Therapy Association.

ISBN-10: 1-56900-217-7
ISBN-13: 978-1-56900-217-9
Library of Congress Control Number: 2006935465

Composition by Grammarians/Laura Johnson Hurst
Printing by Automated Graphics Systems, White Plains, MD

Citation: Stav, W. B., Hunt, L. A., & Arbesman, M. (2006). *Occupational therapy practice guidelines for driving and community mobility for older adults.* Bethesda, MD: American Occupational Therapy Association.

Contents

References 105

Tables, Figures, and Boxes Used in This Publication

■ ■ ■

Acknowledgments

The American Occupational Therapy Association (AOTA) acknowledges the Centers for Disease Control and Prevention, the National Highway Traffic Safety Administration, and the University of Florida for funding support in developing this Practice Guideline.

The authors would like to acknowledge the following individuals who worked with them on the Older Driver Evidence-Based Literature Review:
Paula Bohr, PhD, OTR/L, FAOTA
Karen Buchinger, BSN, MLS
Kathleen Harder, PhD
Amol Karmarker, MS, OT
Joseph M. Pellerito, Jr., MS, OTR
Stacey Scheppens, MS, OTR.

The authors also thank the following individuals for their participation in the development of this publication:
Elin Schold Davis, OTR/L, CDRS
Mary Frances Gross, COTA/L, CDRS
Anne Hegberg, MS, OTR/L, CDRS
Miriam Watson Monahan, MS, OTR, CDRS, CDI
Karen Smith, OT/L
Carol Wheatley, MS, OTR/L, CDRS.

The AOTA Older Driver Expert Panel includes
Elin Schold Davis, OTR/L, CDRS
Mary Frances Gross, COTA/L, CDRS
Linda Hunt, PhD, OTR/L
Dennis P. McCarthy, PhD, OTR/L
Joseph M. Pellerito, Jr., MS, OTR
Susan Pierce, OTR/L, CDRS
Susan Redepenning, OTR/L, CDRS
Wendy Stav, PhD, OTR/L, SCDCM.

■ ■ ■

Introduction

Purpose and Use of This Publication

Practice guidelines have been widely developed in response to the health care reform movement in the United States. Such guidelines can be a useful tool for improving the quality of health care, enhancing consumer satisfaction, promoting appropriate use of services, and reducing costs. The American Occupational Therapy Association (AOTA), which represents nearly 35,000 occupational therapists, occupational therapy assistants, and students of occupational therapy, is committed to providing information to support decision making that promotes a high-quality health care system that is affordable and accessible to all.

Using an evidence-based perspective and key concepts from the *Occupational Therapy Practice Framework: Domain and Process* (AOTA, 2002), this Guideline provides an overview of the occupational therapy process for community mobility among older adults. It defines the occupational therapy process and the nature, frequency, and duration of intervention that occurs within the boundaries of acceptable practice. This Guideline does not include all appropriate methods of care, and it does not recommend any specific method of care as appropriate; the occupational therapist makes the ultimate judgment regarding the appropriateness of a given procedure in light of a specific client's circumstances and needs.

It is the intention of AOTA, through this publication, to help occupational therapists and occupational therapy assistants, as well as the individuals who manage, reimburse, or set policy regarding occupational therapy services, understand the contribution of occupational therapy in treating older adults with driving and community mobility needs. This Guideline also can serve as a reference for health care practitioners, state driver licensing agencies, age-related agencies, transit and transportation authorities, municipal planning organizations, older adults, families and caregivers, health care facility managers, education and health care regulators, third-party payers, and managed care organizations. This document may be used in any of the following ways:

- To assist occupational therapists and occupational therapy assistants in communicating about their services to external audiences
- To assist other health care practitioners, state driver licensing agencies, age-related agencies, transit and transportation authorities, municipal planning organizations, older adults, families and caregivers, and health care facility managers in determining whether referral for occupational therapy services would be appropriate
- To assist third-party payers in determining the medical necessity for occupational therapy
- To assist health and education planning teams in determining the population and community's need for occupational therapy
- To assist legislators, third-party payers, and administrators in understanding the professional education, training, and skills of occupational therapists and occupational therapy assistants (see Appendix A)
- To assist program developers, administrators, legislators, and third-party payers in understanding the scope of occupational therapy services
- To assist program evaluators and policy analysts in this practice area in determining outcome measures for analyzing the effectiveness of occupational therapy intervention
- To assist policy, education, and health care benefit analysts in understanding the appropriateness of occupational therapy services for driving and community mobility services among older adults

- To assist occupational therapy educators in designing appropriate curricula that incorporate the role of occupational therapy related to driving and community mobility among older adults.

The introduction to this Guideline continues with a brief discussion of the domain and process of occupational therapy. This discussion is followed by a detailed description of the occupational therapy process for driving and community mobility among older adults. Next is a description of evidence-based practice as it relates to occupational therapy and a summary of evidence from the literature regarding best practices in driving and community mobility for the older adult population. Finally, appendixes contain additional information about occupational therapists and occupational therapy assistants, the evidence-based literature review, and driving and community mobility among older adults and other resources related to this topic.

Domain and Process of Occupational Therapy

Occupational therapists' expertise lies in their knowledge of occupation and of how engaging in occupations can be used to improve human performance and ameliorate the effects of disease and disability (AOTA, 2002).

In 2002, the AOTA Representative Assembly adopted the *Occupational Therapy Practice Framework: Domain and Process.* Informed by the previous *Uniform Terminology for Occupational Therapy* (AOTA, 1979, 1989, 1994) and the World Health Organization's (WHO; 2001) *International Classification of Functioning, Disability, and Health,* the *Framework* outlines the profession's domain and the process of service delivery within this domain.

Domain

A profession's *domain* articulates its members' sphere of knowledge, societal contribution, and intellectual or scientific activity. The occupational therapy profession's domain centers on helping others participate in daily life activities. The broad term that the profession uses to describe daily life activities is *occupation.* As outlined in the *Framework,* occupational therapists and occupational therapy assistants[1] work collaboratively with clients to promote engagement in occupation to support participation in context or contexts, regardless of the practice setting or population (see Figure 1). This overarching mission circumscribes the profession's domain and emphasizes the important ways in which environmental and life circumstances influence the manner in which people carry out their occupations. Key aspects of the domain of occupational therapy are defined in Box 1. When driving and community mobility are addressed, many terms are used that are drawn from different fields such as driver education, transportation safety, automotive industry, human factors engineering, and occupational therapy. Some terms used in the driving and community mobility practice area are included in Appendix F.

Process

Many professions use the process of evaluating, intervening, and targeting outcomes that is outlined in the *Framework.* Occupational therapy's application of this process is made unique, however, by its focus on occupation (see Figure 2). The process of occupational therapy service delivery begins with the *occupational profile,* an assessment of the client's occupational needs, problems, and concerns, and the *analysis of occupational performance,* which includes the skills, patterns, contexts, activity demands, and client factors that contribute to or impede the client's satisfaction with his or

[1] *Occupational therapists* are responsible for all aspects of occupational therapy service delivery and are accountable for the safety and effectiveness of the occupational therapy service delivery process. *Occupational therapy assistants* deliver occupational therapy services under the supervision of and in partnership with an occupational therapist (AOTA, 2004). When the term *occupational therapy practitioner* is used in this document, it refers to both occupational therapists and occupational therapy assistants (AOTA, 2006).

Figure 1. Domain of Occupational Therapy. This figure is included to allow readers to visualize the entire domain with all of its various aspects. No aspect is intended to be perceived as more important than another.

Note. From "Occupational Therapy Practice Framework: Domain and Process," by American Occupational Therapy Association, 2002. *American Journal of Occupational Therapy, 56,* p. 611. Copyright © 2002, American Occupational Therapy Association. Reprinted with permission.

▨ **Evaluation**

Occupational profile—The initial step in the evaluation process that provides an understanding of the client's occupational history and experiences, patterns of daily living, interests, values, and needs. The client's problems and concerns about performing occupations and daily life activities are identified, and the client's priorities are determined.

Analysis of occupational performance—The step in the evaluation process during which the client's assets, problems, or potential problems are more specifically identified. Actual performance is often observed in context to identify what supports performance and what hinders performance. Performance skills, performance patterns, context or contexts, activity demands, and client factors are all considered, but only selected aspects may be specifically assessed. Targeted outcomes are identified.

▨ **Intervention**

Intervention plan—A plan that will guide actions taken and that is developed in collaboration with the client. It is based on selected theories, frames of reference, and evidence. Outcomes to be targeted are confirmed.

Intervention implementation—Ongoing actions taken to influence and support improved client performance. Interventions are directed at identified outcomes. The client's response is monitored and documented.

Intervention review—A review of the implementation plan and process as well as its progress toward targeted outcomes.

▨ **Outcomes (Engagement in Occupation to Support Participation)**

Outcomes—Determination of success in reaching desired targeted outcomes. Outcome assessment information is used to plan future actions with the client and to evaluate the service program (i.e., program evaluation).

Figure 2. *Framework* Process of Service Delivery as Applied Within the Profession's Domain.

Note. From "Occupational Therapy Practice Framework: Domain and Process," by American Occupational Therapy Association, 2002. *American Journal of Occupational Therapy, 56,* p. 614. Copyright © 2002, American Occupational Therapy Association. Reprinted with permission.

Box 1. Key Terms From the *Framework*

Performance in areas of occupation:

The broad range of life activities in which people engage, including
- Activities of daily living that are oriented to taking care of one's own body, such as bathing (Rogers & Holm, 1994)
- Instrumental activities that are oriented toward interacting with the environment, such as home management (Rogers & Holm, 1994)
- Education that incorporates activities needed for being a student and participating in a learning environment
- Work activities needed for engaging in remunerative employment or volunteer activities (Mosey, 1996, p. 341)
- Play activities that provide enjoyment, amusement, or diversion (Parham & Fazio, 1997, p. 252)
- Leisure activities that people engage in during discretionary time (Parham & Fazio, 1997, p. 250)
- Social participation activities that involve interactions with community, family, and friends (Mosey, 1996, p. 340).

Performance skills:

Features of what one does, not what one has, related to observable elements of action that have implicit functional purposes (Fisher & Kielhofner, 1995). Motor, process, and communication/interaction skills enable people to carry out occupations.

Performance patterns:

Established modes of behavior related to habits, routines, and roles.

Context(s):

The array of interrelated conditions within and surrounding an individual that influence performance, including cultural, physical, social, personal, spiritual, temporal, and virtual dimensions.

Activity demands:

The aspects of an activity, which include the objects, space, social demands, sequencing or timing, required actions, and required underlying body functions and body structure needed to carry out the activity.

Client factors:

Body structures and body functions that reside within the client and that may affect performance in areas of occupation. Body structures are "the physiological functions of body systems (including psychological functions)" (WHO, 2001, p. 10).

Note. From "Occupational Therapy Practice Framework: Domain and Process," by American Occupational Therapy Association, 2002, *American Journal of Occupational Therapy, 56,* pp. 620–626. Copyright © 2002, American Occupational Therapy Association. Adapted with permission.

her ability to engage in valued daily life activities. Therapists then plan and implement intervention using a variety of approaches and methods in which occupation is both the means and ends (Trombly, 1995). Occupational therapists continually assess the effectiveness of the intervention and the client's progress toward targeted outcomes. The *intervention* *review* informs decisions to continue or discontinue intervention and to make referrals to other agencies or professionals. Therapists select outcome measures that are valid, reliable, and appropriately sensitive to the client's occupational performance, satisfaction, adaptation, role competence, health and wellness, prevention, and quality of life.

■ ■ ■

Occupational Therapy Process for Driving and Community Mobility for Older Adults

Driving and community mobility issues occupy a central place in the lives of older adults and their families and friends. The interaction between the changes that take place during aging and a desire by the older adult to age successfully may result in challenges to the older adult's independence in the area of driving. On a policy level, driving and community mobility are becoming increasingly more important given the changing demographics in U.S. society. Currently, 35 million Americans—approximately 13% of the population—are ages 65 or older. By 2020, when the baby boomer generation has almost completely reached retirement, 1 in 5 Americans will be 65 or older (U.S. Department of Transportation, 2003). It also is estimated that by 2030, the number of adults 65 years and older will have doubled (Pike, 2004), and projections indicate that by 2050, the world's population of older people will exceed the population of children (Center for Injury Prevention Policy and Practice, 2002). In addition, older adults are living longer, and over the next 50 years, the population of individuals ages 85 and older is expected to grow faster than any other age group (Federal Interagency Forum of Aging-Related Statistics, 2000).

Driver licensing is, at present, very high among the elderly population, and it is predicted that, by 2012, almost every man and more than 90% of women living in the United States will enter their retirement years as drivers (Rosenbloom, 1999). Older adults are reported to make approximately 85% of all their trips outside the home using a car, either as a driver or passenger (Rosenbloom, 1999). Reports of driving cessation as an independent risk factor of depressive symptoms in elderly people (Berkmon & Tinettin, 1997; Marottoli et al., 1997; Ragland, Satariano, & MacLeod, 2005) point to the central importance of driving a car in the lives of older adults.

All older adults hope for a good life as seniors, often called *successful aging*. Different models have theorized what successful aging, which was originally described by Havighurst (1961) as "getting satisfaction from life," means. Recent research (Phelan, Anderson, Lacroix, & Larson, 2004) has indicated that older adults define successful aging as multidimensional, encompassing physical, functional, psychological, and social health. This view balances the strengths of the older adult with the functional and physical changes taking place.

During the aging process, certain structural and functional changes occur, but there is wide variation in the rate and extent of the changes for the individual older adult. All physiological systems exhibit atrophy, dystrophy, and edema at the cellular levels. These processes are reflected on the functional level in decreased accuracy, speed, range of motion, endurance, coordination, stability, and strength.

Some of the physical changes that affect driving and community mobility occur in the areas of vision, cognition, and mobility. Changes in vision that occur with age include decreased visual acuity, a decrease in night vision, less color sensitivity, and difficulty with the recognition of objects in motion. Glaucoma,

7

cataract, macular degeneration, and diabetic retinopathy are some of the eye diseases that can affect driving. Decreases in speed of process, memory, and problem solving are among the cognitive changes that occur as an individual ages. Changes that affect mobility include decreased strength, less flexibility, changes in posture, and decreased balance reactions. The presence of arthritis and frequent falls also may affect driving and community mobility.

Changes in the social structure also affect the lives of older adults. Divorce, the death of friends and family members, or moves by family members to different geographic locales can have far-reaching effects on an older adult. If an elderly person is living on a limited income, this will determine where he or she can live, the services to which he or she will have access, and the activities in which he or she can participate.

These changes can limit the number and length of trips an older adult can make, because of reductions in strength, endurance, finances, and the ability to get into and out of a car or bus. The changes also can affect the time of day one can drive or travel because of differences in visibility, traffic, noise levels, and the schedules of potential traveling companions. In addition, the age-associated changes combined with health-related issues can result in a higher number of motor vehicle crashes in older adults (Wang, Kosinski, Schwartzberg, & Shanklin, 2003). According to the National Center for Health Statistics (NCHS, 2004), motor vehicle crashes are the second highest cause of injury-related deaths among people older than age 65. Evidence indicates that fragility begins to increase at age 60 and increases steadily with age (Li, Braver, & Chen, 2003).

Compared with other drivers, older drivers have a higher fatality rate per mile driven than any other age group except drivers under the age of 25 (National Highway Traffic Safety Administration [NHTSA], 2003). Not only are drivers ages 75 and older involved in significantly more motor vehicle crashes per mile driven than are middle-age drivers, older drivers are considerably more fragile and have difficulty recuperating after a crash. In 2000, persons over age 65 represented 13% of the U.S. population but accounted for 18% of all traffic fatalities (NHTSA, 2003).

Engagement in occupation is the overarching objective of the occupational therapy. Community mobility, which includes driving, is an instrumental activity of daily living (IADL), one of the areas of occupation AOTA, 2002). *Community mobility* can be defined as "moving the self in the community and using public or private transportation, such as driving, or accessing buses, taxi cabs, or other public transportation systems" (AOTA, 2002, p. 620). Although driving and community mobility are important in their own right, they are especially valuable because they facilitate performance in other areas of occupation, including leisure, work, and social participation. A survey by AARP (2003) asked older adults to list activities that were important for maintaining their quality of life, and the following were rated highly: spending time with family and friends (96%), participating in religious or spiritual activities (82%), and participating in exercise and physical activity (80%). The ability to navigate one's community could potentially be required for participation in all three areas.

Fifty-three percent of respondents to the AARP (2003) survey reported recent difficulty doing something that they needed or wanted to do, such as going for a ride, walking on the beach, making a minor car repair, going to the park with grandchildren, and taking a child to a ballgame. These responses reflect how important community mobility can be to enable older adults to remain independent, maintain a connection with others, and age successfully. According to Pierce and Hunt (2004), individuals move about their world as pedestrians, drivers, or passengers in motor vehicles or on public transportation, or even as users of wheelchairs or scooters, to maintain their relationships with others. Viewed from this perspective, community mobility is an occupation that is essential to personal health and social well-being.

The value of the automobile in society has expanded significantly over time. According to Gartman (2004) and Urry (2004), sociologists have stopped viewing the car as a consumer product and instead now see it as a system of interlocking social and technical practices that have changed society. Sheller (2004) wrote that "Car consumption is never simply about rational economic choices, but is as much about aesthetic, emotional and sensory responses to driving, as well as patterns of kinship, sociability, habituation and work" (p. 222). In all areas of occupation, the tools one uses to develop performance skills and performance patterns are important; however, it is much more difficult to separate the car from the driving experience, because the car has much greater significance than other tools used in the performance of an occupation. For example, driving in the car may be an integral part of an individual's daily routine, and there also may be a social expectation that the husband does the driving while the wife is the passenger. In addition, driving together in a car may be a highlight of a couple's daily routine.

Occupational therapists have been instrumental for more than 30 years in the development and delivery of driver rehabilitation for people with disabilities of all ages and diagnoses. A historical perspective on the role of occupational therapy and driving and community mobility is provided in Appendix E. According to Pellerito (2005), occupational therapists contributed a holistic approach to driver rehabilitation during this time, with the ability to understand those client characteristics needed to encourage participation in driving and community mobility. This approach, in combination with occupational therapists' understanding of the normal aging process and medical diagnoses and their implications, makes members of the profession uniquely trained and positioned to meet the multifaceted needs of the older driver.

Referral

A referral for occupational therapy services for older adults with questionable driving or community mobility ability may be considered based on a client's diagnosis, performance limitations in areas of occupation, or a history of safety issues. Clients with diagnoses that affect functional performance or are progressive in nature may be referred to establish a performance baseline, determine if the impairments in functional per-

formance have extended to the occupation of community mobility, or ascertain methods to extend driving abilities. Providers noticing impairments in areas of occupation such as activities of daily living (ADLs), other IADLs, or social participation may suggest driving and community mobility services to ensure client safety. In addition, a referral to occupational therapy is appropriate when an individual presents as a safety risk due to a history that includes falls, automobile crashes, or getting lost. The need for driving and community mobility occupational therapy services may become apparent at different phases of the aging, disease, or healing process and can come from any point in the community or health care continuum. The sources of referral to occupational therapy services include but are not limited to

- An individual with concerns about an older person's driving and community mobility ability
- Family members or caregivers
- Third-party payers
- Rehabilitation centers and the occupational therapists, physical therapists, speech–language pathologists, recreational therapists, and wellness specialists who work there
- Physicians of varying specialties, including physiatrists, general practitioners, orthopedists, neurologists, ophthalmologists, internists, gerontologists, psychiatrists, and cardiologists
- Optometrists
- Neuropsychologists and psychologists
- Social workers
- Law enforcement agencies
- Traffic court and competency judges
- Attorneys
- Senior and memory disorder centers
- Area agencies on aging.

Evaluation

Occupational therapists perform evaluations in collaboration with the client and based on targeted information specific to the desired outcomes. The two elements of the occupational therapy evaluation are (1) the occupational profile and (2) the analysis of occupational performance (AOTA, 2002). The driving evaluation may take place between a client and an occupational therapist who is either a generalist practicing in a variety of settings or a driving rehabilitation specialist who has the skills and knowledge to provide clients with a comprehensive driving evaluation. Schold Davis (2003) explained that occupational therapists, across a variety of practice areas, may have clients whose disability affects driving or the potential to drive. At the generalist level, occupational therapists evaluate clients' driving subskills and consider the implications of the evaluation. For example, the occupational therapy generalist considers the following:

- Is the client ready to participate in a driving evaluation once discharged from occupational therapy services?
- Have strengths been identified from the occupational performance analysis that suggests the ability to be able to return to safe driving?
- Have impaired skills been identified from the analysis of occupational performance that may affect the ability to drive safely?
- Does the client's occupational profile conclude that there is a desire or necessity to drive?

The occupational therapy generalist further explores driving fitness by checking whether the client's vision and medical conditions meet state guidelines for licensure. Consultation with a local driver rehabilitation service or driver licensing agency may be warranted.

Although occupational therapy generalists are responsible for asking clients whether driving is an occupational performance concern or a goal, they do not evaluate driving competence. Occupational therapy generalists should be knowledgeable in or have resources for at least three additional areas: (1) state driver licensing guidelines (e.g., licensing rules regarding age; vision; and special rulings for medical conditions, such as seizures or dementia), (2) types and availability of driving rehabilitation programs, and (3) alternative mobility resources available within therapists' care systems or their communities. Occupational therapy generalists should exercise the same clinical reasoning skills with driving as they do

when evaluating clients' engagement in other areas of occupation.

Data collected by the occupational therapy generalist may be considered a screening for client driving competency (Schold Davis, 2003). *Screening* is defined as obtaining and reviewing data relevant to a potential client to determine the need for further evaluation and intervention (AOTA, 2005a).

Occupational therapists who are driving rehabilitation specialists have levels of training and knowledge in addition to those of other occupational therapists. These therapists have expertise in targeted evidence-based clinical assessments and on-road assessments. Specialists are experts in driving evaluation and the process of obtaining and interpreting data necessary for intervention and are able to establish protocols to determine driving competence and appropriateness of training as well as to assess a client's ability to use a variety of transportation alternatives (AOTA, 2005b).

An evaluation by an occupational therapy driving rehabilitation specialist includes client information and data gathered through assessments, interviews, and observations. Assessments provide specific criteria on which a performance can be judged acceptable. By breaking down the elements of competency into performance criteria, sufficient data can be collected to demonstrate that an individual can perform to the specified standard in a specific role, such as driving (Association for Driver Rehabilitation Specialists [ADED], 2004).

By using multiple assessment techniques conducted in the clinic as well as on the road, the specialist gathers more data, providing a more solid foundation on which to make a judgment about a driver's competence. Some strategies for assessing driving competencies include client age and diagnosis, the specialist's observation of the client's handling of the vehicle in various traffic environments, the client's self-evaluation and goals, and standardized and nonstandardized assessments (ADED, 2004).

A partnership between the occupational therapy generalist and the specialist may provide the best model for client services. For example, the generalist, through a screening process, identifies a client's need for referral to a driving evaluation and rehabilitation program. On completion of the driving evaluation, the specialist may provide driving rehabilitation or may refer the client back to the generalist for additional occupational therapy services. The generalist may then address impaired performance skills or recommend a follow-up evaluation and intervention plan that result in the design and implementation of an individualized community mobility plan.

Case studies illustrating the occupational therapy evaluation process are presented in Boxes 2 and 3.

Occupational Profile

The purpose of the occupational profile is to determine whom the client or clients are, identify their needs or concerns, and ascertain how these concerns affect engagement in occupational performance. Information can be gathered informally or formally and can be collected during one or more sessions.

Developing the occupational profile involves the following steps:

- *Identify the client or clients.* Although the driver is usually the primary client, a caregiver, physician or other health care provider, or a state licensing agency or law enforcement also may be clients. Most often, therapists evaluate a driver and provide the evaluation results to one or more of the other clients. Therapists also need to know the state driver licensing regulations for reporting client evaluation results and be aware of the AMA's Physician's Guidelines to Driving (Wang et al., 2003). Clients will be better served when all the parameters are known to the evaluator.
- *Determine why the client is seeking services.* Through interviews or checklists, the occupational therapist assists the client in identifying the current concerns relative to the areas of occupation and performance. This is the most critical part of the evaluation. Assessing drivers' insights as to why they are engaged in the driving evaluation will tell the therapist whether intervention is feasible. Clients who lack insight into their capa-

bilities may engage in practices that are less than safe. For example, clients with dementia or other deficits in cognitive functioning lose the mechanism that normally allows people to be aware of their own cognitive abilities. They might undertake activities that are too difficult for them to perform. Furthermore, they are usually unreceptive to the evaluation process and do not believe that they require intervention. This impaired insight is often an obstacle to the rehabilitation process. In general, most clients hope to resume or continue driving, with or without intervention or adaptive mobility equipment. Driving affects engagement in other IADLs (e.g., shopping, visiting friends and family, engaging in various entertainment venues, receiving medical care, engaging in wellness activities, being involved in spiritual traditions). Through an interview, occupational therapists seek information to evaluate how driving influences other activities. The activity analysis in Table 1 presents some demands associated with driving.

- *Identify the areas of occupation that are successful and the areas in which the client is experiencing problems.* On the basis of the client's current concerns, the occupational therapist identifies possible barriers and supports related to occupational performance.
- *Discuss significant aspects of the client's occupational history.* These can include life experiences (e.g., medical interventions, employment history, vocational preferences, responsibilities in the community that require transportation), interests, and previous patterns of engagement in occupations that provide meaning to the client's life. These experiences may shape how the person deals with everyday routines and occupations.
- *Determine the client's priorities and desired outcomes.* Before intervention occurs, it is important that the therapist and the client discuss and prioritize outcomes so that the therapist's evaluation and intervention will match the client's desired outcomes. The therapist may need to refer the

Box 2. Case Study I: Illustration of Occupational Therapy Evaluation

Occupational Profile

Judy Marx, a frail but alert and cheerful woman of 79, has osteoarthritis and osteoporosis that force her to rely on a walker. She had been living at Riverside Meadows, an assistive-care facility, since her husband's death 4 years ago. She does not have any relatives in the area. Although Riverside Meadows provides a van for transportation in the community, Mrs. Marx continued driving her four-door vehicle to activities that include a weekly movie matinee, her long-standing monthly book club, and her volunteer activities at a grade school that she has continued since retiring as a teacher.

Mrs. Marx fell while transferring from the shower. She was taken by the paramedics to the emergency room of the nearest hospital. The X rays of her left hip showed a fracture of the femoral neck and severe osteoporosis of the hip. Mrs. Marx was admitted to the orthopedic ward of Riverside Hospital and underwent surgery for an internal fixation of the fracture. This repaired the break but did not improve her mobility. Mrs. Marx received occupational therapy, which consisted of dressing and bathing aids and training in their use. She was discharged from the hospital and returned to Riverside Meadows.

After recuperating for a month, Mrs. Marx decided to visit her friends at the book club. She attempted to transfer into her vehicle but found that she could not bring her left leg into the vehicle. Using her walker, she returned to her apartment and phoned the nurse practitioner who worked with her physician. The nurse suggested an evaluation by an occupational therapist. Mrs. Marx said that Riverside Meadows had rehabilitation services, so the nurse called to refer Mrs. Marx. The intervention plan for Mrs. Marx continues in Box 4.

Analysis of Occupational Performance

The occupational therapist reviewed Mrs. Marx's records and spoke to her about her goals. While completing an occupational profile, Mrs. Marx discussed her interest in volunteering and participation in social activities. Further discussion revealed contextual barriers as Mrs. Marx reported that the transportation at Riverside Meadows was not available for the types of destinations that were important to her. The occupational therapist continued the evaluation and assessed Mrs. Marx's visual acuity, contrast sensitivity, short-term memory, and ability to perform mental calculations; she found no impairments. During assessments of motor performance and client factors, the occupational therapist noted limited range of motion in Mrs. Marx's lower extremities, left hip pain, and slowness of movement. Mrs. Marx appear to show signs of mild balance deficits, decreased endurance, and impaired coordination of the lower extremities as observed during functional activities.

The occupational therapist believed that adaptive equipment and modified transfer strategies would resolve the problem of transferring in and out of the vehicle, but she wondered if Mrs. Marx had the ability to react quickly to an emergency while driving. The occupational therapist then spoke to Mrs. Marx about a more comprehensive driving evaluation at the hospital's rehabilitation department. Mrs. Marx agreed that fast-moving traffic did overwhelm her at times. The occupational therapist made several referral recommendations to Mrs. Marx's physician to discuss the use of pain medication, to reduce pain; to a physical therapy program, to improve strength, endurance, and coordination; to an occupational therapy driver rehabilitation specialist, for assessment of on-road driving performance; and to the paratransit office of the local bus company, to register for door-to-door transportation services. The intervention plan for Mrs. Marx continues in Box 4.

Box 3. Case Study II: Illustration of Occupational Therapy Evaluation

Occupational Profile

George Conrad, age 83, lives with his wife. He has two daughters who live nearby. His wife no longer drives, and she relies on George for all her transportation needs. Lately, she has been afraid to drive with him because he is impatient, ignores signs, and has had several near-misses. Mrs. Conrad voiced her concern to her daughters, Jean and Sue. Jean suggested that maybe her father should have his vision checked. Sue believes that the problem is more serious, as she has noted that her father is increasingly forgetful and short-tempered and is not as engaged in the family activities as he once was. Mrs. Conrad adds that her husband is interested in seeing friends and participating in hobbies. Sue arranged an appointment for her father with his physician.

The physician suspects early dementia and referred Mr. Conrad to a neurologist. In addition, after hearing Mrs. Conrad's concerns about Mr. Conrad's driving, the physician referred Mr. Conrad to an occupational therapy driving rehabilitation specialist.

Analysis of Occupational Performance

The occupational therapy driving rehabilitation specialist interviewed Mr. and Mrs. Conrad. Mr. Conrad denied the observations that his wife reported. He stated that he does not know why he is having a driving evaluation and complained that it is his physician's mistake. After Mrs. Conrad left the room, and the occupational therapist completed the clinical assessments. Assessments of Mr. Conrad's vision indicate that it is adequate to drive, yet he is experiencing typical age-related changes, including narrowing peripheral fields and decreased contrast sensitivity. The occupational therapy driver rehabilitation specialist found that Mr. Conrad became frustrated with all of the cognitive assessments. He completed the Trail Making Test, Part B, but it took him over 3 minutes to do so (completion time indicating safe driving performance and low risk of crashes is under 90 seconds). He began the Block Design Test but refused to complete it after having difficulty. He also had difficulty saying the months in reverse order during the Short Blessed Exam. Mr. Conrad's motor performance is good, as demonstrated by range of motion within normal limits for all upper- and lower-extremity joints. He had slight limitations in neck rotation to both sides but reported having relied on his mirrors for many years to compensate for an old neck injury. He demonstrated good balance and coordination and was able to complete the Rapid Pace Walk in less than 6 seconds.

The occupational therapy driving rehabilitation specialist noticed the most obvious problems during the on-road test. These include changing lanes without checking traffic, slowing down for a stop sign but not stopping, and making a left turn on a yellow light when he should have stopped.

After the on-road test, the occupational therapy driving rehabilitation specialist recommended that Mr. Conrad not drive until medical options were resolved. The therapist explained to Mrs. Conrad that Mr. Conrad would need supervision for all outings. Mr. Conrad became angry while the therapist explained the results of the driving evaluation. The therapist recommended that Mr. Conrad proceed with his appointment with the neurologist to explore medical options and referred him to a community-based occupational therapist for transportation alternatives and exploration of options for occupational engagement. The intervention plan for Mr. Conrad continues in Box 5.

Table 1. Activity Analysis of Driving

Activity Demand	Driving Demand
Objects and their properties	The vehicle and all components, including the seatbelt, steering wheel, foot pedals, reflective windshield, and keys
Space demands	The driving environment, including the roadway, number of lanes, light conditions, and weather conditions
Social demands	The rules of the road according to traffic laws and courtesy (e.g., allowing a pedestrian to cross the road or another vehicle to enter an intersection)
Sequence and timing	The order in which driving tasks are completed (e.g., shifting the vehicle into gear before accelerating, turning to check behind the vehicle before backing out of a parking space, turning on the directional signal an appropriate distance before turning a corner)
Required actions	The necessary decisions and physical operation of the vehicle (i.e., choosing a route to a store, developing and executing an emergency maneuver, grasping and releasing the steering wheel, turning the steering wheel, moving the right foot from the accelerator to the brake)
Required body functions	The necessary bodily controls for awareness of the driving environment and manipulation of the vehicle controls (e.g., vision to see the roadway and signage, attention to the driving environment, strength to grip the steering wheel, hip range of motion to raise the right foot off the accelerator)

client to additional professionals to achieve these desired outcomes. This also is the appropriate time for the occupational therapist to explore options for alternative transportation with the client.

Analysis of Occupational Performance

Information from the occupational profile is used by the occupational therapist to focus on the specific areas of occupation and the context to be addressed. The following steps are generally included in analyzing occupational performance:

- Observe the client as he or she performs the occupations in the natural or least restrictive environment (when possible), and note the effectiveness of the client's performance skills (e.g., motor, process, communication, interaction) and performance patterns (e.g., habits, routines, roles).
- Select specific assessments and assessment methods that will identify and measure the factors related to the specific aspects of the domain that may be influencing the client's performance. See Table 2 for a summary of these aspects.

- Interpret the assessment data to identify what supports or hinders performance.
- Develop or refine a hypothesis regarding the client's performance.
- Develop goals in collaboration with the client that address the client's desired outcomes. For example, the desired outcome of community mobility may or may not be possible as previously performed.
- Identify potential intervention approaches, guided by best practice and the evidence, and discuss them with the client. For example, the intervention may be driving rehabilitation, or it may be a plan for community mobility provided by an array of resources.
- Document the evaluation process, and communicate the results to the appropriate team members and community agencies. This may include the physician, the licensing agency, and relevant others. Always follow up with the client and significant others.

**Table 2. Examples of Assessments of Occupational Performance for
Older Adults Related to Driving and Community Mobility**

Domain of Occupational Therapy	Sample Assessments Used in Occupational Therapy Practice
Areas of occupation ■ Activities of daily living ■ Instrumental activities of daily living ■ Education ■ Work ■ Leisure ■ Social participation	■ Assessment of Motor and Process Skills (Fischer, 1995) ■ Canadian Occupational Performance Measure (Law et al., 1998) ■ Direct Assessment of Functional Abilities (Karagiozis, Gray, Sacco, Shapiro, & Kawas, 1998) ■ Direct Assessment of Functional Status (Lowenstein et al., 1989) ■ Functional Independence Measure (Center for Functional Assessment Research, 1993) ■ Kohlman Evaluation of Living Skills (Thomson, 1992) ■ Leisure Competency Measure (Kloseck & Crilly, 1997) ■ Leisure Diagnostic Battery (Witt & Ellis, 1984) ■ Leisure Satisfaction Questionnaire (Beard & Ragheb, 1980) ■ Occupational Performance History Interview–II (Kielhofner, Henry, & Whalens, 1989) ■ Occupational Profile ■ Occupational Questionnaire (Riopel & Kielhofner, 1986) ■ Occupational Self-Assessment (Baron, Kielhofner, Lyenger, Goldhammer, Wolenski, 2006) ■ Reintegration to Normal Living Index (Wood-Dauphinee, Opzoomer, Williams, Marchand, & Spitzer, 1988) ■ Self-assessment of leisure interests (Kautzmann, 1984) ■ Structured Assessment of Independent Living Skills (Manchurin, DeBittignies, & Pirozzolo, 1991) ■ Structured observation of performance of activities
Performance skills ■ Motor skills ■ Process skills ■ Communication/ interaction skills	■ Allen Cognitive Level Test (Allen, 1996) ■ Assessment of Motor and Process Skills (Fischer, 1995) ■ Balance Scale ■ Blessed Dementia Rating Scale (Blessed, Tomlinson, & Roth, 1968) ■ Block Design ■ Clinical Dementia Rating (Morris, 1993) ■ Clock Drawing Test (Darwish & Hagin, 1995) ■ COGNISTAT (Neurobehavioral Cognitive Status Examination, Kiernan, Mueller, Langston, & Van Dyke, 1987) ■ Confrontational field testing (Brain Injury Visual Assessment Battery for Adults) (www.visabilities.com) ■ Digit-Span Task (Wechsler, 1997) ■ Hand Disc Perimeter or Vision Disk (www.vernell.com) ■ Hooper Visual Organization Test (Hooper, 1958) ■ Informal coordination tests ■ Letter Cancellation (Uttl & Pilkenton-Taylor, 2001) ■ Map Skills Test ■ Mini-Mental State Examination (Folstein, Folstein, & McHugh, 1975) ■ Motor-Free Visual Perceptual Test–3 (Colarusso & Hammill, 2003) ■ Rapid Pace Walk (Wang et al., 2003) ■ Rey–Osterreith Complex Figure Memory Test and Recognition Trial (Meyers & Meyers, 1995) ■ Rules of the Road Test ■ Stroop Neuropsychological Screening Test (Trenerry, Crosson, DeBoe, & Leber, 1989) ■ Structured observation of performance of activities ■ Symbol–Digit Modalities Test (Smith, 1973) ■ Test of Visual Perceptual Skills–UL (Gardner, 1993) ■ Traffic Signs Test ■ Trail Making Test (Reitan & Wolfson, 2004) ■ Useful Field of View Analyzer (Clay et al., 2005)

(continued)

Table 2. Examples of Assessments of Occupational Performance for Older Adults Related to Driving and Community Mobility *(Continued)*

Domain of Occupational Therapy	Sample Assessments Used in Occupational Therapy Practice

Performance skills *(continued)*	■ Vision testing
	  ■ Color discrimination
	  ■ Contrast sensitivity
	  ■ Depth perception
	  ■ Oculomotor control
	  ■ Visual acuity
	  ■ Visual fields

Performance patterns ■ Habits ■ Routines ■ Roles	■ Activity Configuration (Watanabe, 1968) ■ Driving Habits Questionnaire (Owsley, Stalvey, Wells, & Sloane, 1999) ■ Norbeck Social Support Questionnaire (Norbeck, Lindsey, & Carrieri, 1981) ■ Occupational profile ■ Occupational Role History (Florey & Michelman, 1982) ■ Role Checklist (Oakley, Kielhofner, Barris, & Reichler, 1986)
Context ■ Cultural ■ Physical ■ Social ■ Personal ■ Spiritual ■ Temporal ■ Virtual	■ Accessibility Checklist ■ Canadian Occupational Performance Measure (Law et al., 1998) ■ Driver–vehicle fit assessment (Stav, 2004) ■ Norbeck Social Support Questionnaire
Activity demands ■ Objects used and their properties ■ Space demands ■ Social demands ■ Sequencing and timing ■ Required actions ■ Required body functions ■ Required body structures	■ Accessibility Checklist ■ Driving Habit Questionnaire (Owsley et al., 1999) ■ Structured observation of client driving

Client factors
■ Body functions
■ Body structures
	■ Balance Scale
	■ COGNISTAT (Neurobehavioral Cognitive Status Examination)
	■ Dynamometric measures of grip strength
	■ Geriatric Depression Scale (Brink et al., 1982)
	■ Goniometric measurement of range of motion
	■ Manual muscle testing
	■ Rey–Osterreith Complex Figure Memory Test and Recognition Trials (Meyers & Meyers, 1995)
	■ Sensory testing: Proprioception and kinesthesia
	■ Vision testing
	  ■ Color discrimination
	  ■ Contrast sensitivity
	  ■ Depth perception
	  ■ Oculomotor control
	  ■ Visual acuity
	  ■ Visual fields

Note: This is not an exhaustive list of assessment tools used in occupational therapy in the area of driving and community mobility; instead, it provides an overview of the array of dimensions, methods, and measure incorporated into the evaluation process.

Areas of Occupation

Occupational therapists traditionally evaluate and work with clients to remediate deficits in skills required for driving. Occupational therapists must examine how they can use evidence-based assessments to determine areas of deficiency so that they can then begin interventions that improve the IADLs of driving and community mobility. Occupational therapy's domain centers on helping others participate in daily life activities, some of which may depend on clients' ability to drive. Driving influences and facilitates other IADLs. For example, driving influences the number of trips one can take to see family and friends and one's ability to engage in hobbies and activities outside of the home, and it provides the means to seek and receive nutrition, goods, and services.

Using appropriate assessments and interventions to enable older adults to drive is critical, because driving is increasingly the primary mode of transportation for older adults. It has been shown that those without transportation report decreased life satisfaction (Taylor & Tripodes, 2001) and may become depressed, isolated, and dependent (Marottoli et al., 1997). The ability to remediate client factors helps optimize and prolong older drivers' ability to drive safely, and it increases opportunities for engagement in a range of activities, from everyday ADLs to education, work, play, leisure, and social interactions. Occupational therapists' ability to provide skilled interventions is based on their expertise and knowledge about the screening and evaluation process.

Performance Skills

The driving evaluation includes overt and subtle factors that may affect driving performance. Performance skills, the observable elements of action of an occupation (in this case, driving), can be subdivided into *motor skills, process skills,* and *communication/interaction skills.* For driving and community mobility, motor performance skills include posture, mobility, coordination, strength, and effort. Required process skills include level of energy; knowledge; adaptation; and temporal, space, and object organization. The older adult also needs to be able to engage in the interaction skills of information exchange and the development of relations with others to participate in driving and community mobility. Although difficulties with certain performance skills, such as strength or lack of insight, may be noted at the start of the evaluation process, deficits in other skills, such as getting lost in familiar driving environments or the inability to complete a driving trip because of fatigue and reduced endurance, may be more subtle or not observed at all.

For example, a client with multiple sclerosis may experience fatigue after a shopping trip. Also, a client with Parkinson's disease may experience sudden involuntary movements because of a new problem with medication. In these two examples, an occupational therapist may need to address strategies such as time limits for activities to avoid factors that may negatively affect driving. In a final example, the occupational therapist may not realize that an older client is having difficulty with process and interaction skills until she describes how she interacts with members of her social group to arrange an outing to a restaurant. In this example, the occupational therapist may need to develop a script or written checklist that the client can use when calling her friends to make sure not only that all appropriate information is covered but also that everyone on the list is contacted. Occupational therapists must cover the "what-if" questions that may not surface during the actual evaluation process.

Performance Patterns

Performance patterns are "behaviors related to daily life activities that are habitual or routine" (AOTA, 2002, p. 632); they include habits, routines, and roles. Each is important to driving and community mobility and must be included in a driving evaluation.

Driving habits are the specific, automatic behaviors in which an individual engages. A driving evaluation will determine, for example, whether the client uses a directional signal or mirrors when changing lanes. Routines, established sequences of behavior, provide the structure to enable an occupation.

The occupational therapist needs to examine the roles, or sets of behaviors with socially accepted norms, engaged in by the client. For example, a man may assume the role of driver if a female is in the car. This information is needed for the evaluation, because it will help determine how frequently the client needs to drive, when the activity of driving needs to take place, and whether the client's role as a driver needs to be modified or changed.

Contexts

Occupational therapists acknowledge the influence of cultural, physical, social, personal, spiritual, temporal, and virtual contextual factors on occupations and activities. Factors that support or inhibit performance should be identified during the evaluation process.

Cultural

The evaluation process should include knowledge about each person's cultural beliefs and behaviors. This may result in more inclusive client information. For example, the present belief in prolonging life and independence may be a family cultural belief. An elderly client may be seeking a driving evaluation to continue an independent lifestyle. As another example, husbands who have always been the family driver may not be receptive to allowing their wives to take over the occupation of driving when they are no longer able to drive.

Personal

Personal attributes, such as gender, socioeconomic status, age, and level of education, all factor into the evaluation process. One example is a woman who provides transportation for her friends. She sees herself as a leader and someone who is connected to the community. After an illness, she wants to resume her responsibilities to reaffirm her identity and therefore seeks a driving evaluation. She may not be receptive to being a passenger now instead of a driver. This client has the motivation to engage in an evaluation that may keep her independent.

Physical

The physical driving environment is a critical part of the evaluation process. For example, consider clients who live in rural areas who are often required to merge into two-lane roadways from their driveway. This becomes problematic for drivers with reduced reaction time and information-processing speed. Other contextual factors need to be considered for people living in a suburban or urban environment. For example, if a client has difficulty with glare from the sun, the occupational therapist will need to know the prime driving times for this person. The driving evaluation becomes a means for occupational therapists and clients to explore options for the best routes that promote safer conditions for driving.

Social

The client's social context is important in terms of driving expectations. Older adult communities consist of people along the full spectrum of driving capabilities, ranging from those who are independent and safe drivers to those who are retiring from driving. The social context dictates that clients who are more independent provide transportation to those who are more dependent. This symbiotic relationship exists within the family unit between spouses and within the community among friends and neighbors. The context creates a reliance on the healthier, more independent individuals to serve as transportation providers to access shopping, medical care, and social events. This interdependence is part of the social context and is often the motivation behind wanting to remain a licensed driver.

The loss of a license for a single older adult driver directly affects the occupational engagement of that person. That same license revocation also indirectly hinders the occupational engagement of all individuals who received rides from that person, including his or her spouse, significant other, friends, neighbors, or a stranger participating in a shared-ride arrangement.

When individuals believe they are incapable of meeting life's challenges, they may believe that they are not worthy of happiness and that they are a burden to others who have to provide transportation. Driving clearly affects clients and all others involved in their lives. Clients have reported after they stop driving their social contacts decline (Hunt, 2001):

They [family] may act like it doesn't bother them but it does … takes them away from their own family.

I feel hurried when I ask a family member for help because they have their own commitments to keep.

Your requests have to be kept to a minimum; you limit the things you want to do. (pp. 82–83)

Clients and significant others undoubtedly will face challenges when a driving evaluation results in cessation of driving. It is the responsibility of the occupational therapist to assist clients and significant others with strategies that promote social opportunities.

Temporal

On a large scale, *temporal context* may refer to the time in a person's life span. For older adults, it may signal the time in their lives when another activity becomes difficult to perform, and health care providers, significant others, and clients themselves are seeking advice about the safety or ability to continue driving. Temporal context also may refer to the point in the progression of or recovery from a disease. On a smaller scale, time may figure into the evaluation process, because one needs to evaluate clients at times when they would normally drive. The occupational therapist would need to know whether the client drives at night or during rush hour periods. It also would be important to know how long the person drives each time he or she is on the road.

Spiritual

The *spiritual context* is "the fundamental orientation of a person's life; that which inspires and motivates that individual" (AOTA, 2002, p. 663). This aspect of context reflects the truest essence of the person and draws from intrinsic values, beliefs and goals. Clients may be in touch with their spiritual context by using the time alone in a vehicle as quiet time for reflection. Driving may facilitate engagement within a spiritual context by driving to places of worship or scenic places that nurture the spirit. The strong internal desire to drive or continue driving often times in indicative of a client's

spiritual context and the value placed on autonomy and spontaneity—the goals for independence.

Virtual

A driving simulator is an example of a virtual environment. Simulator use may provide clients with readiness skills before a driving evaluation. Simulators also can offer opportunities for a contextually relevant activity contributing to developing client awareness or insight or may be another tool to evaluate client insight and cognitive skills, such as information-processing speed.

Activity Demands

Determining whether a client may be able to complete an activity depends not only on the performance skills, performance patterns, and client factors but also on the demands of the activity itself. The demands of an activity are aspects of the activity that include the tools needed to carry out an activity; the space and social demands required by the activity; and the skills, body functions, and body structures needed to take part in a given activity. Driving is a complex activity that incorporates most elements of activity demands.

Client Factors

The natural aging process, injuries, and illnesses cause declines in different aspects of client factors, specifically, body functions. The activity demands of driving require that drivers have adequate cognitive, sensory, and motor control of the vehicle and driving environment. Assessment of these client factos can inform the occupational therapist about the client's ability to drive, anticipated client behaviors during the on-road assessment, or elements that should be incorporated into the on-road assessment to challenge the client.

Considerations in Assessments

It is critical that therapists use their clinical reasoning to decide which assessments are selected for each client. This careful selection of assessments will provide the most valuable data and eliminate the tendency to assess every client characteristic. For example, if a client is being evaluated because of a diagnosis of dementia and is physically healthy, then there is no reason for the therapist to spend excessive time assessing muscle strength, range of motion, or sensation. When evaluating older adults, the evaluation process should not be several hours in length, as client fatigue and frustration may confound the results.

Additionally, the evaluation process needs to be based on functional ability that is guided by age or diagnosis. For example, occupational therapists need to be aware of data on types of accidents associated with various age groups (e.g., as a group, older adult drivers have accidents associated with left turns and merging into traffic, whereas teenage drivers have accidents related to high-speed driving). Information about the driver's medical diagnosis also may guide what assessments are chosen. For example, whereas clients with Parkinson's disease may have motor disorders consisting of tremors, the "on–off" phenomenon, and slowness of movement, those with traumatic brain injury may show signs of visual–spatial or behavioral disorders. Although a medical diagnosis may alert an occupational therapist to choose specific assessments, an individual diagnosed with a medical condition may or may not experience measurable functional decline. One person with diabetes may have pronounced visual impairment (e.g., diabetic retinopathy), whereas someone else with another form or stage of the disease might experience little or no visual loss.

Occupational therapists should collect assessment data from a variety of sources, including, but not limited to the client, relevant others, physicians, other therapists who have provided treatment, social workers, the local department of motor vehicles to verify recent accidents or citations, and others who might have knowledge regarding the client's ability to drive.

The role of the occupational therapist on the driving evaluation team is defined by the services offered by the practitioner, the services that are required by the client, the skill mix of the other team members, and the scope of occupational therapy practice as it is defined in the state or jurisdiction where services are being provided.

Assessment Instruments

Some assessment tools are very strong in terms of their psychometric properties, whereas other tools provide valuable qualitative information. As the field of driver rehabilitation is developing, particularly in the emerging practice area of older driver assessment, assessment tools are undergoing rigorous investigation with regard to their utility and ability to predict crashes and driving performance. Therapists are challenged to use careful, educated judgment when selecting tools and interpreting the results in the context of driving. Several assessment batteries with titles or descriptions that include application to driving evaluation may in fact contain only portions of other standardized assessments or unresearched—and not defendable—lists of activities, quizzes, and exercises. Occupational therapists need to use their critical reasoning skills, including knowledge of medical conditions and training in assessment and driving to make decisions about which assessment tools to use.

Occupational therapists must be careful in selecting assessment tools. Many assessments have been associated with driving, such as the Useful Field of View Analyzer (Clay et al., 2005), Trailmaking Test (Reitan and Wolfson, 2004), and Contrast Sensitivity tests. Although some of these tools have limitations in their clinical utility, they may also provide valuable information about the client's performance and behaviors when clinical observations and clinical reasoning are used. For example, during the administration of these tools, a therapist may glean information about a client's problem-solving skills, frustration tolerance, or planning and organization skills.

Reading published articles from the peer-reviewed literature on assessments used in driving and community mobility evaluations will provide important details that may guide the use of specific assessments for individual clients. Occupational therapists should note the following:
- *Diagnosis of the study participants.* Is the assessment valid for other diagnoses?
- *Population of the study.* Is the sample size large enough to justify the recommendations? Were the participants volunteers?

- *Training of the people who collected the data.* Were multiple people collecting the data or providing the training? Was reliability between data collectors or trainers established?

In addition, the reader should have a complete understanding of the circumstances or limitations that might influence the results that were obtained. What were the problems encountered during the research study? What factors were beyond the researchers' control?

Evaluation Based on Valid and Reliable Assessments

The quality of an assessment tool is based on its psychometric properties, or the reliability and validity of the measure. *Reliability* is the extent to which the assessment measure is consistent and free of error. Reliability incorporates not only the structure of the assessment but also what happens when the assessment is administered. Types of reliability include the following (Portney & Watkins, 2000):

- *Test–retest reliability:* Consistency over time if the assessment is administered repeatedly
- *Intrarater reliability:* Consistency of the same rater over more than one occasion
- *Interrater reliability:* Consistency of the measure when two or more evaluators administer the assessment to the same participants
- *Internal consistency:* Consistency of the assessment in measuring the various aspects of the same characteristic.

Although reliability is important whenever one is evaluating an older driver, it takes on additional importance if more than one therapist performs the driving evaluation or if one needs to administer the same test within a short period of time (Hunt et al., 1997b).

Validity refers to the extent to which an assessment measure tests what it intends to measure. According to Portney and Watkins (2000), because a valid measure is relatively free from error, a valid instrument also would be reliable. Types of measurement validity include the following:

- *Face validity* determines if the test seems to measure what it should.

- *Content validity* establishes whether the test assesses the domains it claims to measure; this can be done by a consensus of experts that ensures that the items included in the measure adequately sample the universe of content.
- *Concurrent validity* establishes validity when two measures are taken at the same time, and one is considered to be the gold standard for assessment in a given area.
- *Predictive validity* determines whether a measure predicts future performance on a criterion variable.
- *Construct validity* determines whether an instrument adequately measures a theoretical construct (Portney & Watkins, 2000).

A table created by Korner-Bitensky, Sofer, Gelinas, and Mazer (1998) has identified driving-specific assessments and their related psychometric properties.

The use of validated questionnaires and assessments is a good way to minimize validity and reliability problems, provided that they are administered in an appropriate manner. The following are rules that occupational therapists must use to ensure reliability and validity of assessments:

- Read the directions carefully, and follow the assessment protocols and scripted instructions without exception.
- Complete all sections and items.

On-Road Assessment

In general, occupational therapists and driving clients believe that the on-road assessment is the gold standard for driving evaluation because of its face validity. The on-road assessment is a contextually based test that allows the occupational therapy driving rehabilitation specialist to observe actual driving performance. Administering this assessment is the driving equivalent of assessing a client's ability to perform in the kitchen safely through observation of a cooking task.

The on-road assessment allows the therapist to observe performance over time, in a variety of roadway conditions, responses to different challenges either presented or imposed, and may be a precursor to determining the need for adaptive equipment. While careful consideration is necessary when deciding whether or not to conduct an on-road assessment with clients who have dementia, an on-road assessment should be administered to clients with other diagnoses, as it is a valuable tool in determining fitness to drive.

Benefits of the on-road assessment include the following:

- An assessment of driving is done in a naturalistic environment.
- Real-life perceptual challenges are presented.
- Real-time sensory feedback is given while driving.
- Consequences for negative driving behavior are determined.
- Real-life problem solving is required.
- It is invaluable in making clinical determinations about safety.
- It offers the ability to determine the need for adaptive equipment and to ascertain a client's ability to learn to use that equipment.

On-road assessments can take place in several environments, including on the roadways near a client's residence, on unfamiliar roadways or on a fixed-route or flexible-route course. The course designed for the individual client should reflect the information obtained during the occupational profile and clinical assessment results so that the client can be appropriately challenged according to strengths, weaknesses, and goals. It is important to determine the types of roads and places (e.g., grocery store parking lot, two-lane rural roadway, merge lane onto an interstate highway, neighborhood streets) that the client drives and find locations that simulate these driving demands. Although the on-road driving assessment may be performed in the client's natural environment, the assessment must challenge driving behaviors by including left turns with no traffic control, intersections, merges, and lane changes.

On-road assessments often are performed by an occupational therapy driving rehabilitation specialist; however, other models can be used to administer this test. Programs that include both occupational therapists and occupational therapy assistants may use one individual to conduct the clinical assessments while the other conducts the on-road assessment. Some programs employ a driver educator or driving instructor who conducts the driving assessment from the front seat while the occupational therapy practitioner sits in the back seat and scores the performance. Other programs do not own a vehicle and contract to another occupational therapist or a driving school to administer the test.

In models that incorporate another individual or agency to complete the on-road test, it is essential to develop and maintain a clear line of communication among relevant entities. The occupational therapist who interprets the clinical assessments should communicate to the on-road assessor what is and is not expected during the test, specific maneuvers that should be included based on clinical assessment performance, and challenges that should be presented. The occupational therapist performing the evaluation should receive the on-road assessment results to interpret and synthesize with the history, occupational profile, and clinical assessments to make a final determination about fitness to drive and to develop an intervention plan.

There are several limitations and cautions to be aware of with on-road assessment. Much of the problem has to do with sensitivity and specificity. *Sensitivity* is the ability to detect a problem when the target condition is really present. For example, if a client is impaired and should not be driving, an on-road assessment may not reveal the impairments because of subjectivity of scoring; the inability to control variables such as traffic flow, road conditions, and other drivers' behavior; and the habitual nature of driving. These limitations may increase evaluator error, causing an impaired driver to pass the on-road evaluation (Hunt et al., 1997a).

Hunt et al. (1997a) established reliability and stability of an on-road assessment and noted that the environment contributed to the instability of the on-road assessment. They also reported that driver performance improved when the driver drove behind another vehicle. This condition, called *environmental cueing,* enables drivers to use visual cues from the performance of other drivers to guide their own driving behavior (Hunt et al., 1997a). This supports anecdotal comments from caregivers that drivers with cognitive impairments seek the actions of other drivers to follow the flow of traffic.

Specificity, which is the probability that someone who does not have an impairment will test negative (Portney & Watkins, 2000), also can be a problem with the on-road assessment. Clients may be highly stressed before their evaluation, and some report not sleeping the night before. Older individuals may never have experienced any driver education or a driving "test" in their lifelong history of driving. Stress may contribute to poor performance and therefore facilitate a false-negative outcome. Knowing that someone is evaluating one's performance may negatively affect the performance.

In summary, the on-road driving assessment may be problematic for the following reasons:

- Subjectivity of scoring
- Overlearned skills or the habitual nature of driving a vehicle, which may give a false-positive conclusion, allowing an impaired driver to continue driving
- Inability to control variables such as traffic flow, road conditions, and other drivers' behavior
- Limitations that may decrease the strength of the relationship between the on-road driving assessment and its relationship with neuropsychological assessments.

In addition to the issues noted above, it is important to consider the impact of other factors, such as cost of on-road assessment and related payment as well as programmatic considerations by the institution.

Some suggestions to improve the validity of on-road assessment include the following:

- Setting forth specific behaviors that would alert one to unsafe driving (e.g., missing traffic controls and signs, changing lanes without checking traffic, confusion and lack of problem solving when negotiating traffic, crossing lane lines without awareness, or near-misses requiring a brake intervention by the evaluator)

- Assessing clients during peak traffic times of the day or, if necessary, requiring another on-road assessment if the traffic environment was not challenging for observing appropriate behaviors.

Suggestions to minimize programmatic issues include

- Using all information from the client, caregiver, other health care providers; neuropsychological assessments; and the on-road assessment to make conclusions about fitness to drive rather than placing more weight on the on-road assessment
- Educating hospitals to consider an occupational therapy driving program to be a community service and agree to absorb the additional costs
- Hiring a part-time occupational therapists, as needed, to administer only the on-road assessment, which will reduce costs.

Occupational therapy practitioners who are driving rehabilitation specialists require specialized education to provide clients with an on-road assessment. Each state's licensing agency will regulate qualifications. For example, some states require a degree or certification as a driving instructor to take a client on public roads or require that the driving rehabilitation service be licensed as a driving school.

Evaluation Outcomes

A critical step in the occupational therapy evaluation process is the synthesis of the assessment results and formulation of an intervention plan. In driving rehabilitation, the synthesis culminates with designation of the client's performance and potential for driving into one of three basic categories. This phase sets the future direction of the therapeutic process. Although clients may not remain in a single category for the remainder of their driving longevity, assignment to a single category at the conclusion of the evaluation process is essential to establishing an individualized intervention plan. The categories reflect the client's potential to drive independently and safely and are dependent on the person's underlying performance skills, performance patterns, contexts, and client factors.

The highest performance category is independent and safe performance needing no further intervention.

To be rated at this level, a client must demonstrate adequate motor, process, communication/interaction performance skills, safe contexts in which to perform, and stable client factors while operating a vehicle safely. Safety is a critical component at this level. Individuals who have intact skills and can demonstrate safety on the road may benefit from preventative driver education but do not require occupational therapy services after the assessment. Clients with progressive illnesses such as multiple sclerosis, dementia, or macular degeneration may be assigned to the highest category at the time of the evaluation but need to be reevaluated at designated intervals due to the progressive nature of the disease process to ascertain safety as performance skills and client factors deteriorate.

The second category of potential is the ability to drive safely after therapeutic intervention to improve performance to a maximal level for control of the vehicle and safety. For optimal safety, intervention may focus on the driver, adaptations to the vehicle, or the driving environment. Alternative transportation may be encouraged at this stage as a temporary means for community mobility while the individual is learning to drive using the adaptive equipment. This category suggests that the person has the capacity for improvement in their performance and therefore would eliminate individuals who are in the later stages of progressive illnesses such as Alzheimer's disease. Individuals who may have the potential to improve basic performance skills may be referred back to the occupational therapy generalist for additional treatment. Clients who have never driven before may need therapeutic intervention to learn to drive with gradual or graded learning experiences to learn how to drive for the first time. These clients include older adults who have always depended on a spouse for transportation and now need to take on the responsibility of driving.

The final category of potential includes clients who cannot independently or safely operate a motor vehicle because of visual, motor, or cognitive impairments and do not have the capacity to make improvements. Safety is often the deciding factor in placing clients in this category. A person with good physical control over the vehicle and visual access to the driving environment may not be able to safely engage in driving because of cognitive impairments. The role of safety is particularly important when considering the occupation of driving, because unsafe driving endangers the driver, his or her passengers, and other road users. For the benefit of personal as well as public safety, "the level of independence in task performance may need to be sacrificed for safety" (Hopkins & Smith, 1985, p. 326), and "the physical and psychological benefits of maintaining independence must be weighted against the potential physical damage if an injury occurs." (Arbesman, Campbell, & Rhynders, 2001, pp. 102–103.)

Medical Reporting

Clients assigned to the lowest level of performance should be encouraged to cease driving and receive education related to the legalities of licensure, state identification cards, transportation alternatives, and community resources. Some clients are willing and able to consistently follow the recommendation to stop driving; however, some clients, particularly those with cognitive deficits and impaired insight, have more difficulty in the transition to driving retirement. Clients who do not willingly surrender their driver's license need to be reported to the proper authorities in the state of licensure.

Occupational therapists should be aware of the medical reporting guidelines in the state where they practice as well as neighboring states, if they work near state borders. Medical reporting guidelines include information about the reporting process and filing necessary paperwork. Review of medical reporting guidelines should include identification of

- Parties who may report
- Strength of reporting language—*must* report/*shall* report, *may* report/*authorized* to report
- Level of confidentiality in reporting
- Presence or lack of legal immunity.

Should the client be judged as having potential to drive following training with or without adaptive equipment, the driver licensing agency may require a medical review before resumption of active driving.

Occupational therapists can locate information about medical reporting guidelines in the AMA's *Physician's Guide to Assessing and Counseling Older Drivers* (Wang et al., 2003). The American Association of Motor Vehicle Administrators also sponsors a project aimed at compiling state guidelines for medical reporting. The project maintains a Web site, updated regularly, detailing the guidelines of each state. The report titled "Summary of Medical Advisory Board Practices" can be found at http://www.aamva.org/drivers/drv_AgingDrivers.asp.

Considerations When Evaluating Clients With Progressive Dementia

The community mobility and driving evaluation begins the process of driving cessation for clients diagnosed with progressive dementia, such as Alzheimer's disease. Individuals may become unsafe in the earliest stages of the disease as they lose insight (i.e., fail to recognize) that the dementia is affecting their driving performance. Sometimes it is not dangerous driving behaviors that make them unsafe; instead, it may be the problem of getting lost and confused while driving in familiar environments. Getting lost can have serious consequences, such as driving until there is no longer fuel in the tank and thus risking exposure to the elements, resulting in dehydration, hypothermia, hyperthermia, or death.

Clinical assessments and caregiver reports become valuable measurements for clients with dementia. The on-road assessment is less valuable for determining driving ability for the reasons previously explained. See Table 3 for one recommended approach to evaluating driving for clients with dementia.

The Assessment Hierarchy guides the occupational therapist through the evaluation process. Initially, it was designed to be used with clients with Alzheimer's disease. However, it also can be used with people with a variety of diagnoses such as multiple sclerosis, diabetes, Huntington's disease, Parkinson's disease, and cerebral vascular diseases because it captures key information such as client and caregiver insight. In addition, the hierarchy guides the assessment of cognitive abilities that relate to driving, such as speed of processing information, sequencing, selective attention, and attention switching. Together, the therapist and client progress from assessing concepts understandable to the client such as vision to more abstract assessments. Finally, it includes collecting information on community mobility options, which may be used in the final recommendations provided by the therapist. The focus of evaluation is not to maximize function but to help clients decide on and plan for driving cessation.

Intervention Plan

As a part of the occupational therapy process, the occupational therapist develops an intervention plan that documents the client's goals within an occupational framework, the planned approaches, and recommendations or referrals to others. The plan outlines and guides the therapist's actions and is based on selected theories and frames of reference and the best available evidence to meet the identified outcomes (AOTA, 2002).

The intervention plan will take different directions depending on the outcome of the evaluation, the client's goals, the client's health status, and contextual factors. The plan for a client who presents with stable health status and demonstrates safe, independent performance during the evaluation will be brief and will include approaches to maintain driving safety. The plan for a client with a progressive illness who performs safely during the evaluation will involve education and follow-up monitoring of performance. A more intricate plan will be developed for a client with impairments and less-than-adequate performance during the evaluation; it may include interventions to enhance the person's skills or modification of the task or the environment. A vastly different plan will be developed for clients who perform poorly during the evaluation and do not have potential to improve or benefit from driving specific interventions. A community mobility plan in this situation will incorporate

Table 3. Assessment Hierarchy for Clients With Dementia

Self-assessment

Lacks insight into deficits	Does not self-limit driving activities	Not receptive to alternative options for transportation	Lacks understanding of why the driving evaluation was recommended	Minimizes explanations for problems with driving

Family Assessment

Reports older driver becoming lost on familiar routes	Signs of confusion while driving; difficulty at intersections and merging into traffic	Recognizes that other drivers use evasive actions to avoid crashes; observes other drivers honking at older driver		Has been nervous or fearful as a passenger; does not allow children to drive with driver

Visual Assessments

Visual acuity/near vision	Visual acuity/distance vision	Contrast sensitivity	Depth perception	Visual fields

Visual Processing and Cognitive Assessments

Trail Making Test, Parts A and B (Reitan, 1958)	Short Blessed Test (Katzman et al., 1983)	Traffic symbol recognition (Carr, Labarge, Dunnigan, and Storandt, 1998; Hunt et al., 1993)		For clients with probable dementia: Clinical Dementia Rating Scale (Morris, 1997; Ott et al., 2005)

Knowledge of Alternative Transportation

Cognitive inability to use independent alternative transportation	Accommodations for physical disabilities	Safety and comfort level of using strangers to provide transportation	Availability of family and friends	If still driving, starting the process of letting someone else drive

Road Test

Closed course to establish orientation to the testing vehicle	Progressive traffic interaction	Stop assessment when it is established unsafe		If driver passes, use clinical reasoning when clinical/family assessments show impairments; advise driving cessation (Hunt et al., 1997b)

Follow-up

Determine whether client and family are following the recommendations provided regarding driving cessation or whether the client is to be re-evaluated in 6 months		Determine whether the client is accessing transportation options	Inquire about depression; refer client to primary physician or social services for care	

transportation alternatives and community resources and train the individual and caregivers in the use of the identified resources.

Any of the above-mentioned plans may also include educational resources addressing specific topics such as transporting grandchildren in car seats and planning for driving retirement through choices in housing and proximity to transportation alternatives. The resources and infrastructure to support senior mobility is lacking in most geographic areas. There are tremendous opportunities for therapist advocacy for funding, access, services, or design to enhance driving and community mobility opportunities for the aging population.

Intervention Implementation

The development of goals and intervention methods specific to the topics of older adult driving and community mobility must balance independent performance with safety. The occupational therapist designs interventions that foster engagement and participation in community mobility, an IADL. Although independence and safety in community mobility are primary targets of intervention, therapists should recognize the secondary gains, because enhanced community mobility enables engagement in other areas of occupation, including education, work, leisure, and social participation.

In addition to occupation-based interventions, the therapist might apply a specific theoretical perspective to address driving and community mobility among older adults. In this case, the public health model would be appropriate, because the emphasis is on health promotion and disease prevention for the entire community, incorporating interventions aimed both at the individual as well as the environment.

Within the public health model, the Haddon matrix (Runyan, 1998) is used by professionals in the field of injury prevention to determine the potential causes for an injury. According to the Haddon matrix, the causes of an injury are based on the interaction of the person, the social environment, and the physical environment with the agent, which is the force or substance that causes a change. In the case of the older adult drivers, the older adult is the person; the agent is the car; the physical environment is the infrastructure, which includes roads, lighting, and signage; and the social environment includes policy and community mobility issues. To prevent injuries, a therapist could apply these physics-based concepts related to crash dynamics to determine which is the most appropriate way to avoid injuries to the older adult.

Occupational therapists and occupational therapy assistants, in general, use several approaches to enable clients to meet their goals. These approaches, typically used in combination, are described as follows:

- *Create* or *promote* occupational performance
- *Establish* or *restore* occupational performance
- *Maintain* occupational performance
- *Modify* occupational performance
- *Prevent* deterioration of occupational performance.

Examples of occupational therapy intervention under the rubric of these five approaches as outlined in the *Framework* are provided in Table 4. The types of interventions available to occupational therapists and occupational therapy assistants also need to be considered when determining the most effective treatment plan for a given client. The types of interventions include therapeutic use of self; therapeutic use of occupations and activities, which include occupation-based activity, purposeful activity, and preparatory methods; consultation; and the education process.

Although all types of occupational therapy interventions are used for all approaches, the therapeutic use of self is an overarching concept that should be considered in each therapeutic interaction. Therapeutic use of self is a vital responsibility of the occupational therapist and occupational therapy assistant as well as all the members of the health care team. Perhaps the fundamental attribute required is the ability to listen and understand the gravity of concerns.

The description that follows sets out examples within these approaches and types of occupational therapy intervention for driving and community mobility among older adults (see Boxes 4 and 5; also see Table 5 for case descriptions).

Create or Promote Occupational Performance

Although it is assumed in this approach that the individual does not have a disability in driving or community mobility, occupational therapy practitioners can create opportunities for increased participation in community activities for clients with varying abilities. This approach provides contextual and activity experiences to enhance performance in driving and community mobility among older adults.

Creating strategies involves the design of new tasks that allow for engagement in meaningful occupations, health, and fulfillment of life roles. This strategy is primarily focused on the identification and education regarding community mobility options for

Table 4. Occupational Therapy Intervention Approaches and Examples of Their Use With Driving and Community Mobility for Older Drivers

Approach	Focus of Intervention	Examples of Occupation-Based Goals
Create/Promote: An intervention approach that does not assume a disability is present or that any factors would interfere with performance. This approach is designed to provide enriched contextual and activity experiences that will enhance performance for all persons in the natural contexts of life (Dunn, McClain, Brown, & Youngstrom, 1998, p. 534).	Performance skills Performance patterns Contexts Activity demands	Create skills to use transit systems as an alternative to driving Promote the use of transportation alternatives with regularly scheduled group outing experiences Create a network of community resources to support client's needs after driving cessation Promote community-wide use of transit through simplified use and voucher programs for seniors
Establish/Restore: An intervention approach designed to change client variables to establish a skill or ability that has not yet developed or to restore a skill or ability that has been impaired (Dunn et al., 1998, p. 533).	Performance skills Performance patterns	Restore range of motion and coordination to operate vehicle controls Establish a routine for community mobility for efficient use of transit services
Maintain: An intervention approach designed to provide the supports that will allow clients to preserve their performance capabilities that they have regained, that continue to met their occupational needs, or both.	Performance skills Performance patterns Contexts	Maintain physical agility through participation in a walking wellness program Maintain appropriate medication schedule in coordination with driving schedule Maintain safe and clear walkable communities through collaboration with municipal agencies
Modify: An intervention approach directed at finding ways to revise the current context or activity demands to support performance in the natural setting … [includes] compensatory techniques, including enhancing some features to provide cues, or reducing other features to reduce distractibility (Dunn et al., 1998, p. 533).	Performance skills Performance patterns Contexts Activity demands	Achieve optimal physical control over vehicle steering through installation of a steering device Modify routines and schedules to reduce driving to low-risk/non-rush-hour times Maximize visual access to the driving environment through modification of the driver's seat position in a vehicle Reduce the complexity of left turns by limiting turns to intersections with control signals
Prevent: An intervention approach designed to address clients with or without disability who are at risk for occupational performance problems (Dunn et al., 1998, p. 534).	Performance skills Contexts	Prevent deterioration of driving skills through participation in a driver refresher course Prevent injury during crashes through education and training related to vehicle safety features

individuals who can no longer drive. These options should not be limited to public transportation systems but should include private companies, services affiliated with senior centers, tax-based programs serving municipalities, religious organizations that provide transportation, diagnosis-specific support services, and volunteer programs. In addition, the therapy practitioner should explore service delivery programs for prepared and grocery foods, prescriptions, library services, and so on. Occupational therapy practitioners should use caution when recommending a new situation or context for clients with progressive dementia, as their ability to learn new tasks may be compromised. Before considering transportation alternatives, therapy practitioners must incorporate the client's cognitive status, particularly the client's ability to accomplish new learning, into the decision-making process. Clients with cognitive impairments may have difficulty learning to use new equipment, reading schedules, and negotiating through routes and exchanges.

The process of identifying all potential area resources is time consuming and does require the updating of contact phone numbers and availability of

Box 4. Case Study I: Illustration of Occupational Therapy Intervention

After analyzing the results of the occupational profile and assessment, the occupational therapist determined that several different intervention approaches would be appropriate to address Mrs. Marx's community mobility needs.

Create Approach

The occupational therapist was concerned that Mrs. Marx's social contacts had been severely limited by her lack of transportation to her usual activities. The occupational therapist explored ways that Mrs. Marx could stay connected to her activities and social contacts while the underlying problems that impaired her ability to drive were being addressed. The occupational therapist identified transportation alternatives to the grade school for her volunteerism. A taxi drove Mrs. Marx to the school, and a teacher gave her a ride home. She continued to use the taxi and transportation from the teacher even after she improved her strength and mobility. Mrs. Marx decided she enjoyed the conversations with the teacher on the way home. The therapist also identified a door-to-door transportation alternative to bring Mrs. Marx to her weekly movie and book club meeting and assisted in the application process to access these services. Mrs. Marx found that the ride-sharing provided an additional venue for reducing her isolation and supporting socialization.

Restore Approach

The therapist recommended that Mrs. Marx discuss with her physician the use of pain medication to reduce pain and physical therapy to improve strength, endurance, and coordination. Mrs. Marx did receive a pain prescription and anti-inflammatory drug to address medical conditions causing impairments. Furthermore, she improved her stamina and reaction time through an exercise program. The occupational therapy driving rehabilitation specialist to whom Mrs. Marx was referred also provided training to improve Mrs. Marx's driving skills and self-confidence.

Maintain Approach

The combined efforts by the occupational therapy generalist as well as the occupational therapy driver rehabilitation specialist supported Mrs. Marx's mobility with her own vehicle and transportation alternatives. These efforts had a secondary effect, which maintained Mrs. Marx's engagement in occupations of volunteering, socializing, and leisure interests.

Modify Approach

Although Mrs. Marx was able to operate her vehicle adequately, she had difficulty entering and exiting it. The occupational therapy driver rehabilitation specialist provided Mrs. Marx with adaptive equipment, specifically, a leg lifter and a swivel seat to maximize independence in car transfers and a cushion for increased comfort and height.

Prevent Approach

The prescribed adaptive equipment changed Mrs. Marx's sitting position in her car and altered the relationship between her body and the vehicle's safety features. To prevent injuries, the occupational therapy driver rehabilitation specialist analyzed Mrs. Marx's position to ensure sufficient foot contact with the foot pedals, maintaining a safe distance from a deploying airbag, and proper positioning of the seat belt. The therapist adjusted the height, angle, and forward position of the driver's seat to ensure adequate distance from the airbag and raised the shoulder anchor of the seat belt to allow the shoulder belt to cross Mrs. Marx mid-clavicle.

Box 5. Case Study II: Illustration of Occupational Therapy Intervention

Mr. Conrad's impending driving cessation due to cognitive deficits necessitates the establishment of other means of mobility within the community as well as identification of occupations to help maintain his overall health and well-being. To achieve these general goals, the community-based occupational therapist used numerous intervention approaches.

Create Approach

The occupational therapist completed a thorough occupational history with Mr. Conrad to identify occupations that are or have been meaningful to him during his life. The therapist then used a lifestyle redesign model (Mandel, Jackson, Zemke, Nelson, & Clark, 1999) to capture those meaningful occupations and facilitate Mr. Conrad's engagement. The therapist discovered that Mr. Conrad enjoys building model airplanes as well as flying them and fostered this activity between Mr. Conrad and his grandson. The therapist also identified reminiscence and card groups for seniors in the community recreation center in Mr. Conrad's town. The occupational therapist arranged transportation services for Mr. Conrad to get to the community recreation center and set up meeting times to participate in these groups with his friends. In addition to transportation to the community center, the therapist identified a local transportation service that has companions, drivers, and schedulers trained in dementia and aging issues. This door-to-door service is available to transport Mr. and Mrs. Conrad to medical appointments, grocery shopping, social visits, and other necessary errands.

Maintain Approach

One of Mr. Conrad's assets is his physical health. Understanding his need to rely on this asset, the occupational therapist recommended an aquatics exercise program at the community recreation center to maintain his physical health. This program offers transportation through the center and has qualified aquatic therapy instructors as well as volunteers from the local health professions college to provide one-on-one assistance to participants needing additional physical or cognitive guidance.

Prevent Approach

Mr. Conrad's condition is likely progressive in nature, and his community mobility will become more and more restricted over time. To prevent social or occupational disengagement, the occupational therapist worked with the Conrads to identify optimal living environments in anticipation of the time when Mr. Conrad will need more assistance. The occupational therapist helped the Conrads explore continuous-care communities that offer a range of health and independent-living situations, a variety of on-site activities, and transportation services while remaining in close proximity to their daughters.

services; however, once compiled by city, county, region, or other designation, this is a valuable resource to clients who can no longer drive.

The federal government supports such efforts, as indicated in the report *Safe Mobility for a Maturing Society: Challenges and Opportunities* (U.S. Department of Transportation, 2003), which recommends a role identified as a *mobility manager*. A mobility manager serves as a case manager specializing in community mobility, which includes access to community resources to provide for continued occupational engagement despite an inability to drive.

Examples of interventions using the Create/Promote approach include the following:

Table 5. Case Descriptions of Occupational Therapy Interventions for Driving and Community Mobility

Case Description	Occupational Therapy Driving Considerations	Driving Prognosis and Occupational Therapy Intervention[a]
George, age 79, is married and has a retinal detachment.	• Crashes or near-misses related to impaired visual access to the driving environment caused by decreased right visual field. • Poor attention to signage on the side of the retinal detachment due to decreased visual field. • Decreased or ceased driving may result in limited access to health care, socialization, and transportation of his wife.	Continued ability to drive with periodic assessment of visual fields. May eventually need intervention to learn adaptive strategies such as head turning and use of mirrors or adaptive mirrors to compensate for visual field loss. Awareness of the deficit is critical.
Sarah, age 67, is a hospital volunteer coordinator who recently underwent coronary artery bypass grafting surgery.	• Risk for sternal disruption following median sternotomy. • Decreased endurance to tolerate driving for extended periods of time. • Limited upper-extremity strength and range of motion following surgery. • Social withdrawal and lack of meaningful engagement resulting from being away from volunteer experience.	May resume driving 4 weeks following surgery as long as there are no surgical complications and cognition is intact. A driving evaluation is indicated if the client presents with cognitive changes.
Joan, age 63, is a grandmother who had a stroke 2 weeks ago who has primary custody of her grandchildren.	• Motor impairments that may interfere with Joan's ability to enter or exit and to control a vehicle. • Sensory deficits that may limit her visual access to the driving environment or ability to feel the vehicle controls. • Cognitive deficits that may impair Joan's ability to attend to driving and make safe judgments negotiating through the roadways. • Joan's ability to care for her grandchildren and meet their needs.	Temporary driving cessation is recommended until neurological recovery has occurred. A driving evaluation is indicated once her progress has stabilized to determine her ability to drive and the need for adaptations. Joan will likely benefit from adaptive equipment to compensate for her hemiplegia, and she may need assistance with child passenger seat management.
Max, age 83, has Parkinson's disease.	• Motor involvement specific to tremors and difficulty initiating movements may impair Max's ability to operate a motor vehicle. • Cognitive declines associated with the disease progression may limit Max's ability to make quick, safe decisions. • Peak medication times may increase Max's ability to capitalize on periods of improved motor control.	During the very early stages of a progressive neurological disorder such as Parkinson's disease, Max may be able to drive safely. However, Max and his family and friends will need to plan for the eventual need to cease driving. Periodic reassessments of performance are indicated every 6–12 months.
Carlos, age 71, has been taking antihypertensive medication for years to control his high blood pressure; he currently has a cold and is taking an antihistamine.	• Antihypertensive side effects can include lightheadedness, dizziness, fatigue, sedation, confusion, insomnia, and nervousness. • Central nervous system side effects of the antihistamine include sedation and psychomotor impairment. • Carlos's ability to attend to the driving environment and manage the presented challenges may be impaired. • Carlos may attempt to engage in his daily routine without recognition of the effects of medications on his performance and abilities.	Carlos is able to drive but should do so only after discussing medication side effects and interactions with his physician or pharmacist. Carlos will need to be educated about the possibilities of side effects and the influence on his abilities. He also should delay driving until he is aware of how his body will react to these medications and their combination.

(continued)

Table 5. Case Descriptions of Occupational Therapy Interventions for Driving and Community Mobility *(Continued)*

Case Description	Occupational Therapy Driving Considerations	Driving Prognosis and Occupational Therapy Intervention[a]
Marie, age 74, is a widow whose husband passed away 2 months ago and who has been diagnosed with situational depression.	▪ Marie is taking a new medication and is not aware of or accustomed to the side effects. ▪ She may be very tired during the day due to sleeplessness at night. ▪ She may be experiencing cognitive or motor symptoms that could impair driving. ▪ She may be at risk for suicidal ideation, and driving could be hazardous for her and other road users. ▪ She is at risk for isolation and decreased engagement in other meaningful activities.	Once Marie has been cleared of suicidal ideation and is accustomed to the side effects of her medications, she can continue driving safely.
Dorothy, age 62, is an elementary school teacher with insulin-dependent diabetes mellitus.	▪ Unstable blood glucose levels with periods of hypoglycemia and hyperglycemia. ▪ Vision impairments related to diabetic retinopathy if blood glucose levels are not maintained. ▪ Sensory deficits in the lower extremities related to diabetic neuropathy if blood glucose levels are not maintained. ▪ Dorothy is at risk for interruptions of her work-related activities and routine if driving difficulties arise.	Dorothy can drive as long as she maintains control of her blood glucose levels. She should have periodic assessments of her vision and sensation to identify diabetic-related complications. She may eventually need a driving evaluation and adaptive equipment to compensate for decreased lower-extremity sensation.
John, age 82, is a widower who dates frequently and recently underwent surgery for a right total hip replacement.	▪ John may have difficulty entering/exiting vehicles while observing total hip precautions, particularly bucket seats and low vehicles. ▪ Operation of the foot pedals may be impaired due to decreased strength, range of motion, coordination, reaction time, and sensation in the right lower extremity. ▪ He may experience interruptions in engagement in socialization and sexual expression if his driving ability is hindered.	John should temporarily cease driving for at least 4 weeks following surgery and should exercise caution when driving for 8 weeks following surgery until he returns to his baseline function.
Herbert, age 91, has a history of peripheral vascular disease and is the only person in his cohort of friends with a driver's license.	▪ Light touch, deep pressure, proprioception, and kinesthesia may be impaired in the lower extremities and prevent accurate operation of the foot pedals. ▪ Limitations in driving will not only affect Herbert's engagement in the community but also that of his friends, as he is the primary driver.	Herbert should have a thorough driving evaluation to determine his fitness to drive. He may benefit from adaptive equipment to compensate for the unreliability of his lower extremities to operate the foot pedals.
Brenda, age 66, is undergoing chemotherapy and radiation for breast cancer following a mastectomy.	▪ Brenda may experience motor or cognitive side effects of the chemotherapy or radiation. ▪ Antiemtic medication to help with feelings of nausea may cause sedation, blurred vision, headaches, confusion, or dystonia. ▪ She may have difficulty operating the vehicle controls, including the gear selector and steering wheel, due to pain or strength and range-of-motion limitations from the mastectomy.	Brenda should refrain from driving while experiencing side effects of chemotherapy, radiation, and medications. She also should use caution when driving while under the influence of pain medication. Brenda should cease driving until she is aware of the side effects of these medications. She may require therapeutic intervention to increase the strength and range of motion of her effected upper extremity.

[a]Time-related driving recommendations are based on Wang et al. (2003).

- *Identification of transportation alternatives.* The alternatives identified should meet the client's specific needs for community mobility while taking into consideration the client's performance skills, performance patterns, contexts, and the activity demands of the identified services. Occupational therapy practitioners should draw directly from the occupational profile to determine the client's need for mobility in the community and access to programs and services. Choosing transportation alternatives necessitates that the practitioner consider the activity demands of the transportation options, such as scheduling an appointment in advance, waiting for a ride in outdoor conditions, the distance between home and pick-up and drop-off points, the need to count money, and physically accessing the ride. The final selection needs to be based on the demands of the activity and the client's ability to meet those demands. On a community level, occupational therapy practitioners should collaborate with agencies providing transit or other transportation services to promote elder-friendly services through sensitivity training for drivers and schedulers, large-print schedules, assistive technology on buses, and other programs to facilitate service use.
- *Facilitation of registration for transportation services.* Many transportation services provide the supports necessary for clients but include consideration of eligibility criteria as well as a lengthy, complicated application and approval process. Occupational therapists and occupational therapy assistants should assist clients in the application phase and help with verification of need as required. Occupational therapy practitioners also should inquire as to the availability of a voucher program or prepayment plan to eliminate the physical, visual, and cognitive demands of money management during travel.
- *Travel training for clients in the use of transportation alternatives.* Clients not accustomed to transit systems or other transportation programs will benefit from an orientation to the service as well as training in the naturalistic context. Practition-

ers should gradually withdraw assistance and support during use of transportation services. To conserve resources, practitioners should inquire with the local transit and paratransit agencies regarding the presence of travel training programs. In addition, independent-living centers throughout the United States, Canada, and other countries offer travel training to people with disabilities, including older adults. Access to the locations and contact information for Independent Living Center offices can be found at http://www.ilusa.com/links/ilcenters.htm.
- *Coordination of service delivery, such as Meals on Wheels or prescription delivery.* For many clients, setting up transportation services will not completely satisfy their daily needs. Service delivery can supplement the need to travel into the community. Programs such as Meals on Wheels (http://www.mowaa.org/) offer an alternative to using transit to shop at the grocery store. Clients will be benefit from improved nutrition compared with the food they can carry themselves because of limitations due to weight and perishability when using transit. Clients who are capable of using transportation alternatives may appreciate the convenience of prescription delivery or library book-lending by mail. Practitioners should identify all available community resources and supports and maintain a list for use with individual clients who may be interested.
- *Education related to social programming within the client's community.* Often in small communities or in those designed for older adults, there are many opportunities for engagement in activities within the community that do not require driving or transit. For example, large retirement communities typically offer theater, dining, bingo, card games, and social events in the clubhouse on the community property, eliminating the need to drive or to be transported. Occupational therapy practitioners should promote the client's participation in such programming, as it may create a new outlet for occupational engagement without the need to drive.

■ *Promotion of walking and bicycling programs.* Walking and bicycling are both health-promoting activities that serve as positive alternatives to driving. In addition to the physical benefits, there are socialization benefits if walking or bicycling are performed in groups. Occupational therapists working in the community can facilitate the development of such groups and encourage participation by senior members of the community. Careful consideration should be paid to the location of the programs to ensure safety and accessibility.

Establish or Restore Occupational Performance

This approach is directed to restoring or remediating function that approximates levels before the onset of the disease or deterioration. Strategies are focused entirely on the person and are geared toward building or remediating deficits (Dunn, Brown, & McGuigan, 1994). This approach uses occupation as the end result and places sole emphasis on restoration of performance skills, performance patterns, and client factors. The possibilities for remediation are not absolute for all skills, and therapists must consider the type and cause of the each deficit area before attempting remediation. Areas of weakness that are progressive, such as impaired sensation caused by neuropathy or visual loss due to macular degeneration, do not warrant attempts at remediation. Occupational therapy practitioners

should consider that restoration efforts do not have to be performed by the occupational therapy driving rehabilitation specialist and are often best accomplished with the help of occupational therapy generalists or other team members.

Examples of intervention using the Establish/Restore approach are given in Table 6.

Maintain Occupational Performance

This approach is used in occupational therapy intervention to provide supports that will allow clients to preserve their performance capabilities and prevent deterioration of function. This is often achieved through driver refresher courses, which provide didactic or hands-on experiences related to defensive driving, strategies to enhance visual awareness of the environment, and information about current trends and policies. Another approach used to maintain occupational performance is self-assessment, which allows drivers to be aware of their skills while deterioration due to age and illness may be taking place. This awareness results in the confidence to continue driving safely, alter driving habits or patterns, or seek skilled services to maintain community mobility through remediation or adaptation.

Examples of interventions using the Maintain approach include the following:
■ *Walking wellness program to maintain balance and agility.* Participation in a walking program can

Table 6. Examples of Intervention Using the Establish/Restore Approach

Problem	Restore Strategy
Decreased range of motion	Self range-of-motion program, exercise program, other therapeutic intervention[a]
Decreased strength	Exercise program, other therapeutic intervention[a]
Decreased coordination	Coordination exercise program, other therapeutic intervention[a]
Decreased visual acuity	Change in corrective lenses, cataract removal surgery[b]
Decreased visual awareness	Vision training program to increase awareness of the deficient field[a]
Decreased contrast sensitivity	Cataract removal surgery[b]
Decreased arousal	Medication change or reschedule[b]
Decreased attention	Cognitive retraining program to increase attention to multiple stimuli simultaneously[a]
Decreased memory	Medication change[b]
Decreased executive functioning	Cognitive retraining to improve safety by exploring compensation strategies for problem solving and reasoning skills[a]

[a]In preparation for driving, to maximize the client's ability to operate a vehicle and access and process the environment.
[b]Will require collaboration with a physician or pharmacist.

help maintain blood flow, range of motion, strength, agility, and the endurance necessary during driving.

- *Participation in an older driver safety course* (e.g., American Automobile Association, National Safety Council, AARP). Older driver safety courses offered in a classroom setting typically incorporate education related to aging and its effect on driving, defensive driving strategies, positioning of mirrors, a self-assessment, and open discussions. Participation in an older driver safety course benefits the driver through automobile insurance discounts as well as awareness of age-related deficits that necessitate adaptations in driving.

- *Participation in a driver refresher course.* Driver refresher courses are more active and participatory than older driver safety courses. Participants are able to drive in the naturalistic environment while receiving real-time feedback from the instructor. These courses are typically offered through established driving schools or larger entities such as the National Safety Council.

- *Completing a self-assessment.* Many self-assessments are available through state and national government entities as well as through private organiza-tions at the state and national level. Self-assessments, such as the American Automobile Association's RoadWise Review, serve as a tool to maintain a driver's ability through periodic measures of skills used in driving. These measures, used intermittently, are valuable tools to monitor the effect of a driver's aging and illness on performance. Caution should be used when recommending such tools, and they are to be used for self-awareness and screening rather than as a determinant of driving safety.

- *Maintaining medication schedule with timers and medication boxes to allow for consistent medication consumption.* Older adults are consumers of almost one-third of the prescription medications sold in the United States (Avorn, 1995). Occupational therapy practitioners should help clients identify patterns in performance associated with peak medication times. Client and caregiver education is necessary for individuals with notable performance changes due to medication (e.g., clients with Parkinson's disease who have decreased rigidity when medications take effect) to capitalize on peak medication times so that the client can schedule driving during those times. Strategies should be implemented to maintain medication schedules for optimal performance.

Modify Occupational Performance

The Modify approach adapts current circumstances to facilitate occupational performance. This is accomplished by adapting the task, the environment, and the individual's approach (Dunn et al., 1998). Modifications are aimed at changing the context or the task to make engagement in that activity possible (Dunn et al., 1994). The modification does not attempt to restore function to premorbid levels but aims to facilitate optimal engagement at the current level of function. In general, people with degenerative diseases benefit from this approach by compensating for limitations through education about compensatory strategies and adaptive techniques, use of environmental modifications, and adaptive equipment. Therapists should use caution when recommending a new situation or context for clients with progressive dementia, as their ability to learn new tasks may be compromised.

In addition to modifying the task, the method of engaging in the task, or the environment, the occupational therapy intervention plan commonly includes education. This education incorporates explanations for specific driving and mobility techniques; adaptations to automobiles and other transportation vehicles; and current information about the disease process, as well as resources for the client, family, and others.

Contextual Modifications

Modifying contextual factors results in improved performance by adapting or changing the context to better match the person's skills and abilities. The Modify strategy assumes that the status of the client is constant and cannot be restored and uses a more supportive context to improve performance. The client can change the physical or temporal contexts in which driving and community mobility are performed by incorporating education with active and consistent follow-through. Modifying the context may include altering the routine of driving to include safer traffic or lighting conditions or changing a route to avoid high-traffic areas. For modification to be successful, the client must make a commitment to be vigilant in observance of the altered context. If the client has a cognitive impairment, therapists should question the client's ability to consistently adhere to the modifications.

Activity Demand Modifications

Modifying the task results in improved performance by adapting or changing the task to better match the person's skills and abilities. Modifying the tasks assumes that, because the status of the client cannot be improved, a more supportive approach to the task must be used for improved performance. Adapting the vehicle or using compensatory strategies are examples of modifications to the task. Vehicle modifications provide an alternate method of entering and exiting the vehicle, sitting in the vehicle, or operating the vehicle controls. Similar to modifying the context, successful modification requires client commitment for consistent use of the modification. If the client is cognitively impaired, then therapists should question the client's ability to learn to use new modifications or to consistently observe the modifications. Examples of interventions using the Modify approach are presented in Table 7.

Adaptive Equipment

Deciding which equipment to recommend and writing the prescription are critical steps in the client's transition toward independent driving (ADED, 2004). The equipment described in Appendix B used for vehicle operation, such as steering devices, accelerating/braking devices, and secondary controls, should be prescribed by an experienced occupational therapy driving rehabilitation specialist. The occupational therapy generalist should refer to an occupational therapy driving

rehabilitation specialist when there are client concerns related to vehicle operation. The occupational therapy generalist may have concerns related to joint protection or coordination and is capable of recommending adaptive equipment, such as adaptive key-holders. After completing a driver vehicle fit assessment, the occupational therapy generalist may suggest adaptive equipment to facilitate transfers (e.g., a swivel seat) or optimize positioning in the vehicle with cushions. More complex adaptive equipment, particularly that which involves vehicle operations, requires a referral to an occupational therapy driving rehabilitation specialist.

There are a variety of adaptive equipment choices, both in terms of type and manufacturer, so occupational therapy driving rehabilitation specialists should be familiar with the options and purchase samples of each instrument for use in the driving program vehicle. The most obvious option for adaptive equipment should be tried first, but the occupational therapy driving rehabilitation specialist should remain open to other devices, because the most obvious is not always the best choice for a particular client.

For example, a client with a right lower-extremity amputation may very easily be independent with a left-foot accelerator. In many cases, this simple choice may be a quick and easy transition for the driver. In addition, if a client has poor coordination in the left lower extremity or onset of peripheral neuropathy in the left lower extremity, using the left leg for vehicle operation is not a safe alternative. In these cases, hand controls would be a better choice. A client's personal comfort or choice may be the deciding factor in some cases. A client requiring the use of a spinner knob with a completely intact and functional hand may prefer the feel of a single post attachment as opposed to a knob, strictly for comfort reasons.

Final decisions about adaptive equipment should be made only after the client is observed using the equipment while driving. Once the adaptive equipment has been chosen, the therapist must write a prescription to provide specifications for type of equipment; manufacturer, if necessary; additional features; and installation instructions. Detailed prescriptions are used as a road map for equipment dealers to

Table 7. Examples of Interventions Using the Modify Approach

Problem	Modify Strategy
Decreased range of motion	Modify vehicle with additional mirrors to compensate for limited neck rotation
Decreased contrast sensitivity	Drive during light traffic hours only, night driving and avoid driving in the rain
Decreased memory	Limit destinations for travel
Decreased attention	Modify routes to include only low-traffic roadways
Decreased reaction time	Travel on low-traffic roads, avoid highways and rush hour
Wheelchair dependent; cannot transfer	Modify a van allowing for vehicle control from the wheelchair secured to the floor with a lift into the van
Unable to transfer into driver's seat	Modify driver's seat with seat that rotates and projects out of the vehicle
Unable to use right lower extremity functionally	Modify the vehicle with a left-foot accelerator or hand controls
Unable to operate vehicle ignition	Modify the vehicle with a button ignition, or modify the keychain for leverage

Note. Adaptive equipment choices are not absolute for any client and should be tried along with other equipment for best fit and function with the client's abilities, limitations, needs, and vehicle.

generate cost estimates, for correct installation, and as a means for inspection by the equipment dealer and the therapist at the follow-up equipment inspection. Mastery of the adaptive equipment should be attained during training sessions on the driving program's vehicle, and equipment should not be installed until the client is ready for discharge to independent driving with adaptive equipment. It is recommended that the occupational therapist wait until just before the client's discharge to write a prescription, because clients may have the equipment installed and practice without supervision if the prescription is written early in the therapeutic process.

A prescription written with details ensures that installed equipment represents exactly what the client had achieved competence in while using the program's vehicle. An example of a comprehensive prescription should read as follows:

- Drive Master Push–Pull hand control with horn and dimmer switch mounted on the left side
- Steering device with a V-grip installed at the 4 o'clock position with a small base and quick-release grip.

Therapists using adaptive strategies should be prepared to provide training to introduce the client to the equipment, master understanding and operation of the equipment, and help the client safely use the equipment in all driving situations that he or she will encounter. Training sessions should allow the person sufficient time to become accustomed to the adaptive equipment and use the equipment without conscious effort while driving on the roadways. After the equipment has been installed in the client's own vehicle, occupational therapy driving rehabilitation specialists must conduct a checkout of the client and the equipment to ensure accuracy of the prescription, proper installation in the vehicle, and the client's ability to use the equipment.

Prevention of Future Deterioration of Occupational Performance

Occupational therapy intervention also is designed to provide supports to prevent acceleration in the deterioration of function. Although preventing disease progression is outside the domain of occupational therapy, preventing or slowing deterioration in occupational performance is the unique contribution of occupational therapy intervention. This is achieved through provision of equipment, support, and education. Empowering the client and family to use and build on strategies already in place will assist in preserving performance related to driving and community mobility.

Prevention strategies are designed to prevent the occurrence or evolution of maladaptive performance by addressing the person, the context, and the task (Dunn et al., 1994). These strategies are accomplished largely through continued driving practice, education related to driving longevity, and prevention of injuries or problems in the future by avoiding crashes. Many of these prevention strategies are related to driver–vehicle fit and should be instituted regardless of skill level or health status. Other prevention strategies are related to driving behaviors and also should be used by all drivers regardless of health status or independence.

Population-based interventions provide strategies to improve health, support performance, and prevent negative outcomes for communities and larger groups. Occupational therapy practitioners working with a community may use the Prevent intervention approach. These strategies may be directed toward educating drivers and passengers or toward the design of vehicles and communities. Interventions directed toward people as vehicle occupants may be accomplished through health fairs, community presentations, or participation in driver–vehicle fit screening programs. Prevent strategies aimed at vehicle design may involve consulting with vehicle manufacturers regarding elder-friendly controls or access and use of vehicle safety features to reduce injuries. Therapists working with community design professionals or municipal planning organizations can impart their knowledge about older road user risks and roadway design recommendations from the *Highway Design Handbook: for Older Drivers and Pedestrians* (Staplin, Lococo, Byington, & Harkey, 2001) to reduce injuries and fatalities community wide. A comprehensive summary of this handbook can be found in Appendix D. Examples of the Prevent approach are given in Table 8.

Intervention With Clients With Progressive Dementia

When working with clients who have Alzheimer's disease and their families, the first goal is to find solutions for community mobility that maintains the client's identity, roles, and occupations within his or her cultural and environmental domains. This requires a willingness to consider the client's personal situation in shaping recommendations regarding driving fitness, options for training, and recommendations for mobility options.

It also is important to emphasize that unescorted trips into the community are no longer safe and that a client identification bracelet may be needed as a safety measure (Hunt, 2005).

The intervention plan consists of the following referrals:

- *Social services*—What is available?
- *Occupational therapist/psychologist*—Assessing feelings about the self with respect to the problem, enlisting the help of someone who cares, rewarding the self or being rewarded by others for not driving, acknowledging that change is part of the life cycle.
- *Community services*—Alzheimer's centers/associations, agencies on aging, city and county governments, religious affiliations.
- *Physician*—Monitor depression; monitor medication, monitor progression.

Finally, the occupational therapist must have a system in place for follow-up to verify that the plan for transportation is effective. If there are problems, then more intervention is appropriate (see Table 3). Appropriate interview questions to detect problems may include the following:

- Is the client still driving?
- Is the plan for transportation working?
- Is the client abnormally sad since he or she has ceased driving?
- What was the outcome with the licensing agency?
- Has the client been re-evaluated by the physician?

Allowing the individual with dementia to continue to drive places both the driver as well as the other road users at risk, because even mild cases of dementia may pose a serious safety risk (Dubinsky, Stein, & Lyons, 2000).

Reimbursement

Both federal and state laws, as well as the activities of key professional organizations, influence delivery of and payment for occupational therapy services related to driving and community mobility. In the United States, the individual receiving services most often pays for driver evaluation and intervention. In general, specialized driver rehabilitation services are

Table 8. Examples of Interventions Using the Prevent Approach

Prevent Strategy	Desired Result
Wear both lap and shoulder part of seat belt	<ul><li>Prevents ejection from the vehicle</li><li>Provides "ride-down" of energy forces from crash</li><li>Prevents head and upper-body impact with obstacles and steering wheel</li><li>Prevents "submarining" under steering wheel onto floor</li></ul>
Sit 10–12 in. (25–30.5 cm) away from the airbag	Allows space for airbag deployment at 200 mph
Position head rest at ear level or higher and 2.5 in. (6.4 cm) or less from back of head	Prevents excessive backward head excursion in a crash
Tilt steering wheel toward chest, not face	Allows airbag to deploy into chest, avoiding face injuries
Position rearview mirror to encompass entire rear window	Allows maximal visual access to the rear driving environment
Position sideview mirrors with minimal view of vehicle sides	Allows maximal visual access to the side-rear driving environments
Allow 3 seconds following distance behind vehicles	Maximizes available stopping distance
Stop at red lights where driver can see rear tires of vehicle to the front touch the road	Reduces chance of a second collision if driver is rear-ended
Turn left at intersections with a left turn signal	Avoids high-risk left turn maneuvers
Hold steering wheel at 4 o'clock and 8 o'clock positions	Avoids facial injury from airbag propelling arms/hands into face
Seat children younger than age 12 in the back seat	Avoids possible fatalities from adult-intended airbag deployment

not currently considered covered services under Medicare benefits; however, there are a limited but growing number of states in which the Medicare carriers will reimburse for all or part of driver rehabilitation services. The Veterans Administration system provides driver rehabilitation services to veterans at select locations nationwide. State vocational agencies, Medicaid, workers' compensation, and private insurers may cover driver rehabilitation services and vehicle modification. (AOTA, 2005b, p. 667)

Many clients or their family members place value on driving rehabilitation services and are willing to assume the costs associated with services when there is no third-party reimbursement.

Examples of suggested billing codes for evaluations and interventions related to driving and community mobility are provided in Appendix G.

Intervention Review

Intervention review is a continuous process of re-evaluating and reviewing the intervention plan, the effectiveness of its delivery, and the progress toward targeted outcomes (AOTA, 2002). Re-evaluation may involve re-administering assessments or measurement tools (instruments) used at the time of initial evaluation, a satisfaction questionnaire completed by the client, or questions that evaluate each goal (Berg, 1997; Minkelm, 1996). Re-evaluation normally substantiates progress toward goal attainment, indicates any change in functional status, and directs modification to the intervention plan, if necessary (Moyers, 1999). This phase of invention culminates in the final determination of the client's ability to drive independently and safely and successfully negotiate another means of community mobility or adjust the intervention plan and continue accordingly.

Outcome Monitoring

The occupational therapist should regularly monitor the results of occupational therapy intervention to determine the need to continue or modify the intervention plan or to discontinue intervention, provide follow-up, or refer the client to other agencies or professionals. Medical reporting should be included in outcome monitoring for occupational therapy practitioners practicing in states where it is allowed. Medical reporting is important to monitor during the driver rehabilitation process, because responsibility or accountability may be shared across disciplines (e.g., occupational therapy, psychology, medicine) if a client continues to drive when it is not medically indicated.

Outcome monitoring is particularly important for clients with progressive diseases such as Parkinson's disease or Alzheimer's disease. These clients may present with safe and independent driving or community mobility performance at the time of the initial evaluation or after a course of intervention. However, their level of performance may deteriorate as their disease progresses because of impaired motor or cognitive functioning. A timeline for a return visit for the monitoring of performance should be established at the time of discharge to re-evaluate safety and performance as the disease progresses. This continued monitoring will allow the individual to drive as long as possible, prolonging independence and putting off the inevitable need to cease driving until necessary on the basis of driving performance rather than diagnosis.

Documentation

Occupational therapists and occupational therapy assistants should document their services in the areas of evaluation, intervention, and outcomes (AOTA, 2002). Recommendations related to driving restrictions and cessation should be documented and communicated to team members and caregivers. This documentation should be completed "within the time frames, format, and standards established by the practice settings, agencies, external accreditation programs, payers and AOTA documents" (AOTA, 2005a, p. 664). Occupational therapy documentation meets four purposes:

1. It articulates the rationale for the provision of services and their relationship to the client's outcomes.
2. It reflects the therapist's clinical reasoning and professional judgment.
3. It communicates information about the client from an occupational therapy perspective.
4. It creates a chronological record of client status, occupational therapy services provided, and client outcomes. (AOTA, 2003)

The following types of documentation may be completed for each client, as required by law, the practice setting, third-party payers, or some combination of these:

- Evaluation or screening report
- Occupational therapy service contacts
- Occupational therapy intervention plan
- Progress report
- Prescription/recommendation for adaptive equipment
- Re-evaluation report
- Discharge or discontinuation report. (AOTA, 2003)

Readers should refer to the *Guidelines for Documentation of Occupational Therapy* (AOTA, 2003) for specific report contents and fundamental elements of documentation.

Discontinuation and Discharge Planning

Planning for discharge begins at the time initial occupational therapy services are discussed and is based on a determination of independence and safety as well as realistic expectations for community mobility. Discontinuation should take place when the client has achieved established goals, reached full potential, or both. The achievements in performance indicating readiness for discontinuation of services should be established at the time of discharge planning and incorporate contributions from the client, family or caregiver, and other providers involved in the services, including physicians, vision specialists, case managers, and state licensing agencies, as applicable.

Discharge dispositions may include independent driving, transition to transit or paratransit services, or planned monitoring of performance for clients with progressive illnesses. Incorporated into the discharge planning should be recommendations for community services, alternative transportation, or service delivery to complement adapted driving.

Follow-Up

After the client is discharged from occupational therapy services, additional intervention may be needed at a later date. This may be necessary if the client's health declines, the client recovers from a medical condition, medical interventions alter the client's ability to drive, the client ages, the driving context changes, or adaptive equipment needs to be upgraded or adjusted. In some cases, clients may perform well at the time of the initial evaluation, but the aging or disease process may have caused performance changes, thus warranting additional services. Clients undergoing medical interventions such as new medications, cataract surgery, or an amputation may benefit from additional services. Changing contexts (e.g., moving to a new community) may influence performance, because clients do not perform in the same way in differing contexts. Clients moving to new neighborhoods or municipalities may need assistance learning to modify performance in the new context to maintain independence. Advances in technology, old adaptive equipment, or disease progression may justify the need for additional services to allow clients to use the most efficient adaptations for independence. Therapists should maintain an open relationship with clients after discharge so that clients feel comfortable seeking assistance for additional intervention when necessary.

■ ■ ■

Evidence-Based Practice

Why Evidence-Based Practice?

One of the greatest challenges facing health care systems, service providers, public education, and policymakers is to ensure that scarce resources are used efficiently. The growing interest in outcomes research and evidenced-based medicine over the past 30 years, and the more recent interest in evidence-based education, can in part be explained by these system-level challenges in the United States and internationally.

In response to demands of the cost-oriented health care system in which occupational therapy practice is often embedded, occupational therapists and occupational therapy assistants are routinely asked to justify the value of the services they provide on the basis of the scientific evidence. The scientific literature provides an important source of legitimacy and authority for demonstrating the value of health care and education services. Thus, occupational therapists, other health care practitioners, and educators are increasingly called on to use the literature to demonstrate the value of the interventions and instruction they provide to clients and students.

What Is an Evidence-Based Practice Perspective?

According to Law and Baum (1998), *evidence-based occupational therapy practice* "uses research evidence together with clinical knowledge and reasoning to make decisions about interventions that are effective for a specific client" (p. 131). An evidence-based perspective is based on the assumption that scientific evidence of the effectiveness of occupational therapy intervention can be judged to be more or less strong and valid according to a hierarchy of research designs and an assessment of the quality of the research.

AOTA uses standards of evidence modeled from standards developed in evidence-based medicine. This model standardizes and ranks the value of scientific evidence for biomedical practice using the grading system in Table 9. In this system, the highest levels of evidence include those studies that are systematic reviews of the literature, meta-analyses, and randomized controlled trials. In randomized controlled trials, the outcomes of an intervention are compared to the outcomes of a control group, and participation in either group is determined randomly.

The evidence-based literature review presented here includes Level I randomized controlled trials; Level II studies, in which assignment to a treatment or a control group is not randomized (cohort study); and Level III studies, which do not have a control group. Thus, for the purposes of this review, only Levels I, II, and III studies are included.

Best Practices in Older Driver Intervention: Results of the Evidence-Based Literature Review

Focused questions were developed for the evidence-based literature review on older adult driving using a public health approach (Christoffel & Gallagher, 1999). The questions were based on the areas in the Haddon matrix (Runyan, 1998). As mentioned previously, injury prevention requires many components in which the older adult is the person; the agent is the car; the physical environment is the infrastructure, which includes roads, lighting, and signage; and the social environment includes policy and community mobility issues. An expert panel reviewed the intervention questions that were developed to correspond to each area. The following four questions resulted:

Table 9. Levels of Evidence for Occupational Therapy Outcomes Research

Levels of Evidence	Definitions
Level I	Systematic reviews, meta-analyses, randomized controlled trials
Level II	Two groups, nonrandomized studies (e.g., cohort, case control)
Level III	One group, nonrandomized (e.g., before and after, pretest–posttest)
Level IV	Descriptive studies that include analysis of outcomes (e.g., single-subject design, case series)
Level V	Case reports and expert opinions that include narrative literature reviews and consensus statements

Note. Based on Sackett (1986).

1. *The person:* What is the evidence for the effect of interventions to address cognitive, visual, and motor function; driving skills intervention, self-regulation/self-awareness; and the role of passengers and family involvement in the driving ability, performance, and safety of the older adult?

2. *Policy and community mobility:* What is the evidence for the effect of policy and community mobility programs (e.g., licensing regulations, alternative transportation, walkable communities, education, pedestrian programs) on the participation of the older adult?

3. *The infrastructure:* What is the evidence for the effect of modifications of the infrastructure of the physical environment (e.g., roadways, signage, lighting) on the driving ability, performance, and safety of the older adult?

4. *The automobile:* What is the evidence for the effect of automobile-related modifications on the driving ability, performance, and safety of the older adult? This would include changes by the industry that enhance or hinder the driving ability, performance, and safety of the older adult.

Search terms for the review were developed by the project coordinator in consultation with the review authors and with an advisory group of occupational therapists and an occupational therapy assistant with expertise in driving. A medical research librarian conducted all searches to confirm and improve search strategies. Search terms used for all questions included the following: *elderly, older driver, aging, automobile driver, automobiles, traffic safety, automotive engineering, automobile driver simulators, automobile driver examination, driving behavior, motor vehicles, vehicle operation, vision tests, roads and streets, highway markings, traffic signals, signage, glare effects, pavements, illumination, public transportation, communities, physical mobility, environment, transportation, transportation needs, pedestrians, headlights, braking, vision aids, glare, sensory aids, instrument displays, visual environment, highway safety, driver education,* and *traffic accidents.* In addition, a filter based on one developed by McMaster University (http://www.urmc.rochester.edu/hslt/Miner/digital_library/evidence_based_resource.cfm) was used to narrow the search to research studies. The medical librarian and the coordinator of the project discussed the searches and findings to ensure that key articles or areas of research had not been overlooked.

The search consisted of peer-reviewed literature published between 1980 and 2004, and the databases searched included Medline, TRIS online, Ergonomics Abstracts, PsycINFO, Society for Automotive Engineers, EiCompendex Engineering, EiCompendex Plus, Ageline, Sociofile, and CINAHL. For the infrastructure question, the search consisted of peer-reviewed literature published from 1999 through 2004, and the databases searched included TRIS online, Ergonomics Abstracts, EiCompendex Engineering, EiCompendex Plus, and Medline. Information before 1999 was taken from the *Highway Design Handbook: For Older Drivers and Pedestrians* (Federal Highway Administration, 2001), because this document provided guidelines for the highway design for communities across the United States.

Consolidated information sources, such as the Cochrane Database of Systematic Reviews, were included in the search. These databases are peer-reviewed summaries of journal articles and provide a system for clinicians and scientists to conduct 66 evidence-based reviews of selected clinical questions and topics. Published reports, such as those from the Transportation Review Board, also were included in the review, and bibliographies of selected articles were reviewed for potential articles. Exclusion criteria for the review included the following: presentations, conference proceedings, journal articles and reports published prior to 1980, dissertations, and articles from non-peer-reviewed journals.

The review author for each focused question and the coordinator of the project reviewed the articles according to their quality (i.e., scientific rigor, lack of bias) and levels of evidence. Guidelines for reviewing quantitative studies were based on those developed by Law (2002) and colleagues to ensure that the evidence is ranked according to uniform definitions of research design elements.

- *Level I* studies included systematic reviews, meta-analyses, and randomized controlled trials.
- *Level II* studies included two-group nonrandomized studies, such as cohort and case control studies.
- *Level III* studies were one-group nonrandomized studies, such as before-and-after and pretest–posttest designs.
- *Level IV* and *Level V* studies (e.g., descriptive studies, case reports, case series, expert opinions) and dissertations, book chapters, and conference proceedings were not considered for the review.

Thirteen thousand abstracts were reviewed for the 4-question search, and 56 articles met the inclusion and exclusion criteria for the questions. Twenty-six were Level I studies, 22 were Level II studies, and 8 had Level III research designs.

The review of the evidence consists of descriptions of selected studies identified in the evidence-based literature review, appraisals of their strengths and weaknesses based on the study design and methodology,

and their findings relevant to the provision of driving and community mobility–related intervention with older adults. These articles were chosen if the studies either included occupational therapy within the intervention or were within the scope of occupational therapy practice and included interventions to the person, community mobility, the infrastructure, or the automobile to support or improve older driver performance. Articles including policy analyses related to driver licensing also were included in the review. All studies identified by the review, including those not specifically described in this section, are summarized and cited in full in the evidence tables in Appendix C. Readers are encouraged to read the full articles for more details.

The articles/studies were appraised using a critically appraised paper (CAP) format. The CAP consisted of a description of the study, an appraisal of its strengths and weaknesses based on the study design and methodology, and the findings relevant to the provision of driving and community mobility–related intervention with older adults. The article was chosen if the study either included occupational therapy within the intervention or was within the scope of occupational therapy practice and included interventions to the person, community mobility, the infrastructure, or the automobile to support or improve older driver performance. Except as noted below, all review authors were occupational therapists with expertise in the area of driving. In addition, they had the ability to review research literature from an evidence-based perspective.

The process of completing the CAPs was different for each question. For the person, policy, and community mobility questions, for example, the CAPs were written by the reviewers of the focused question. A human factors consultant with expertise in ergonomic issues of older adult driving and a graduate student completed the CAPs for the infrastructure question. The car question was completed by the review author in conjunction with a graduate student. The coordinator of the project reviewed each article and the completed CAP to look for unanswered questions and discrepancies in interpretation of the results and to ensure that the implications were clear.

Review authors for the car, person, and policy and community mobility questions also completed the critically appraised topic (CAT), or summary and appraisal of the key findings, clinical bottom line for occupational therapy practice and study limitations of all the articles included in the review for each question. An occupational therapist who also is a human factors engineer completed the CAT for the infrastructure question. The CATs were reviewed by the coordinator of the project and AOTA staff to ensure quality control.

Interventions to the Person

The evidence-based literature review question asked "What is the evidence for the effect of interventions to address cognitive and visual function, motor function, driving skills intervention, self-regulation/self-awareness, and the role of passengers and family involvement in the driving ability, performance, and safety of the older adult?"

The studies examined in the review focusing on interventions for the person included 3 that examined the effect of visual training, 1 that studied a physical exercise program, 1 that tested the effect of training on a simulator with a navigational system, and 2 that inquired about the impact of passengers on crashes. The evidence provides mixed support for visual training to improve driving with similar contradicting support for passengers in the prevention of crashes. The review supports both home exercise programs for head and neck flexibility to improve visual access of the driving environment and ultimately improve control of the vehicle and navigational systems to promote less erroneous driving.

Mazer et al. (2003) compared the effectiveness of a visual retraining program using Useful Field of View (UFOV) with traditional visuoperception treatment in a Level I randomized clinical trial. All participants in the study had had a stroke within 6 months of the study and had driven before the stroke. Mazer et al. (2001) attempted, in a Level III study, to determine whether UFOV affected actual driving performance by assessing driving after UFOV training. Of the 97 participants who began the study, 84 completed the posttest driving evaluation, with 41 in the UFOV group and 43 in the visuoperception group. The results indicate that there was no difference between groups for failing the on-road evaluation. When the analysis was limited to right-sided lesion, however, participants in the UFOV intervention group were almost twice as likely to pass the on-road evaluation as participants in the control group. This study was limited by the lack of a pre-training driving assessment.

The effect of speed-of-processing (UFOV) training was examined in a Level I randomized clinical trial by Roenker, Cissell, Ball, Wadley, and Edwards (2003). Cognitive training using the computerized Visual Attention Analyzer was compared with driving simulator training (Doron Precision System). Participants in both groups had a minimum of 30% total reduction on the UFOV measure. A low-risk reference group was also included for comparison. Although the driving rating of both intervention groups improved across testing sessions, the UFOV group improved on dangerous driving maneuvers, whereas the simulator-training group improved on turning into the correct lane and proper signal use. At 18 months, the effect of the UFOV persisted, but the effects of the simulator training did not. The study was limited by lack of cognitive evaluation of participants before the study began.

Training older adults who had a stroke and consequent impaired visual attention also was explored by Klavora et al. (1995). In this Level III before-and-after study, a Dynavision apparatus was used to improve performance on several measures of psychomotor ability, such as response time and anticipation time using a behind-the-wheel driving test as the outcome measure. The 10 participants in the study with onset of a stroke between 6 and 18 months before the study had marked visual and attention difficulties when driving and had previously been assessed as unsafe to drive. The results of this study indicated a statistically significant difference for divided and selective attention but not for processing speed. On the second behind-the-wheel assessment, 6 of 10 (60%) participants earned a rating of "safe to resume driving and/or to receive on-road driving lessons," and 4 were assessed as "unsafe to drive at this time." This was compared to an expected rate of frequency for safe assessments of 24% from an historical cohort. The ability to generalize the results of this study to other impaired older adults was limited by the lack of an actual control group and the inclusion of younger adults in the study population.

Ostrow, Shafron, and McPherson (1992) evaluated the effects of an 8-week range-of-motion home exercise training program to improve head and neck flexibility. Participants in the experimental group of this Level I randomized clinical trial improved on trunk rotation to the right and shoulder flexibility and were significantly more likely to have improved on handling position and observing while driving. There was no statistically significant difference between groups in terms of changes in the average number of days driven per week or average number of miles driven per week.

Llaneras, Swezey, Brock, Rogers, and Van Cott (1998) evaluated the effectiveness of a variety of design and education approaches to compensate for age-related changes in commercial vehicle drivers in a Level I randomized controlled trial. Interventions included the use of the Simulated Prescriptive Auditory Navigational System (SPANS), which provided prescriptive routing information in the form of auditory commands versus traditional paper-based maps; training on visual search and scanning patterns; comparison of drivers with and without an on-board advanced auditory warning system; comparison of drivers with an automatic transmission versus drivers with a manual transmission; and a control group with no intervention. Outcome measures included number of missed turns, number of navigational queries, and time to complete the 10-mile (16-km) course; visual search and mirror checks; manipulation of vehicle during curves; executing turns; and speed adjustment. Results indicated that drivers equipped with SPANS made fewer navigational errors and inquires than drivers who relied on paper-based maps and directions. In addition, drivers exposed to the visual search and scanning training program had better monitoring per-formance as measured by visual search and mirror check scores. Drivers provided with an auditory warning had significantly higher detection rates than drivers without the advanced warning system, and drivers whose trucks were equipped with automatic transmission had better performance during curves than their counterparts equipped with the manual transmission. The study was limited by the use of a driving simulator that makes it difficult to generalize the findings to actual on-road vehicle performance. In addition, participants in the experimental group received all four interventions, which may make it difficult to determine which effects could be associated with a given intervention.

Vollrath, Meilinger, and Kruger (2002) analyzed the influence of the presence of passengers in a Level II cohort study using a German database of motor vehicle crashes involving at least two vehicles. The presence of passengers in crashes in which the driver was at fault was compared with crashes in which the driver was not at fault. The results indicated that passengers were protective at all ages, and the protection was strongest for drivers ages 50 years and older. The positive effect of passengers was attenuated, however, when driving at night, in slow and standing traffic, and at crossroads. This study was limited because single-vehicle crashes were excluded. In addition, the difficulty in discriminating between individuals who are at fault and not at fault in a crash may have limited the ability to assign to study conditions accurately.

Hing, Stamatiadis, and Autman-Hall (2003) also examined the role of passengers and crash involvement in a Level II quasi-induced exposure methodology. The authors reported that drivers older than age 75 are even more likely to cause a crash with two or more passengers when they are traveling on curves, grades, and two-lane roads. This risk was decreased however, when driving with no passengers or one passenger at night. This study differs from Vollrath et al.'s (2002) study because all crash involvement was included. Because this study is based on information from a crash database, it does not include factors such as eye health and other components of aging that could affect driving ability.

Interventions Related to Community Mobility

The evidence-based literature review question asked "What is the evidence for the effect of policy and community mobility programs (e.g., licensing regulations, alternative transportation, walkable communities, education, pedestrian programs) on the participation of the older adult?"

Few studies specific to the effectiveness of transportation alternatives as a means for older adults to remain mobile within the community have been conducted. The following study supports an integrative model involving older adults, families, and other stakeholders in program development to maintain elder mobility within the community.

Freund (2002) developed and tested an innovative transportation program, the Independent Transportation Network, that was designed to meet the community mobility needs of older adults by including seniors needing transportation, family members concerned about aging relatives, and the businesses that derived revenue from older consumers. Either older adults or their adult children paid for transportation, and businesses contributed to the financial support of the service. The network used both program employees and volunteers as drivers and a centralized dispatching system. The results of this Level II study revealed that rides to participating merchants were greater in the experimental group. A follow-up survey reported overall satisfaction with the program by merchants as well as the older adult study participants. This study is limited by the lack of a cost–benefit analysis and randomization of groups.

Interventions Related to Driver Licensing

The studies examined in the review focusing on policy related to driver licensing included one study that focused on a restricted licensing program and studies investigating driver license renewal policies. The evidence supports restricted licensing programs to decrease crashes and traffic violations. The studies reviewed support license renewal policies that include one or more of the following: vision testing, in-person renewal, or medical review, depending on age. The collective review of these studies suggests that a graduated increase in renewal criteria as drivers progress from old to older-old may be beneficial in reducing crashes.

Marshall, Spasoff, Nair, and Walraven (2002) evaluated the effectiveness of a restricted license program by comparing the rates of crashes and traffic violations among restricted drivers in Canada to the rates in the general driving population. This Level II cohort study also compared the crash and traffic violation rates before and after driver restrictions were imposed to further examine the impact of the program. The analyses revealed that restricted license holders not only were less likely than drivers with unrestricted licenses to have been involved in a crash (83% vs. 75%), but they also had significantly lower traffic violation rates. With both driving and licensing restrictions imposed, there was a significant decrease of 0.2 crashes per 1,000 drivers per week after the restrictions were imposed, with a relative rate reduction of 12.8%. Analysis of weekly traffic violation rates 4 years before and after imposition of restrictions revealed that a combination of driving and license restrictions significantly decreased traffic violations 0.2 per 1,000 drivers after the restrictions were imposed. This study was limited by the inability to control for driving exposure and a lack of measurement of driver compliance with restrictions. In addition, the data captured only insurance-claimed crashes, which is not indicative of all driving incidents.

Hakamies-Blomqvist, Johansson, and Lundburg (1996) evaluated the safety effect of age-based medical screening on drivers in Finland and Sweden in a Level II cohort study. They compared the crash rates in Sweden, which has no age-related screening or medical review associated with license renewal, to those in Finland, which has strict medical–legal screening associated with license renewal. In Finland, the right to hold a license after age 45 is conditional, as drivers must pass a medical and vision examination every 5 years to renew their license. At age 70, the license expires, and people who want to continue to drive must pass a medical review and submit a new application. Renewal periods shorten after age 80. The two countries vary on licensing rates, with

44.2% drivers ages 70 and older in Sweden licensed and only 14.6% of people the same age licensed and maintaining their driving licenses in Finland. The crash and fatality rates between the countries were similar, with no statistical significance reported. The fatality rate of unprotected road users, including pedestrians and bicyclists, however, was more than twice as high in older adults in Finland than in Sweden. This study was limited because nonfatal crashes were not included in the analysis.

Grabowski, Campbell, and Morrisey (2004) examined whether state driver licensing renewal policies beyond vision testing were associated with fatality rates among older drivers. They studied all traffic fatalities of persons ages 65 and older in the contiguous United States that were reported to the Fatality Analysis Reporting System for the 11-year period of the study. License renewal policies were examined across states, including guidelines related to in-person renewal, vision tests, and road tests. Other factors were identified to control for state speed limits, seat belt laws, blood alcohol limits, and administrative license revocation. In an analysis of older drivers across states, the data revealed that states with in-person renewal had lower fatality rates for drivers ages 85 and older; drivers ages 65 to 74 had lower fatality rates in states with vision tests. A comparison of older and younger driving cohorts indicated that states with in-person renewal had lower fatality rates for drivers ages 85 and older. There was no relationship, however, among vision testing, road tests, and varying lengths of renewal periods and fatality rates of older drivers. This study was limited because nonfatal crashes were not included in the analysis.

Shipp (1998) examined the impact of vision relicensing policies on traffic fatalities in the United States in a Level II cohort study. The study used the Fatality Analysis Reporting System data for a 3-year period and compared fatalities in states with vision relicensing policies to those without the policy. The results suggest that state-mandated vision testing as part of the license renewal process may enhance traffic safety and reduce the economic burden of fatal crashes. For the period studied, 1989 through 1991, an additional 222 older fatalities may have been prevented, saving $31 million in the 8 states without vision testing. Although this study provides comprehensive information on fatalities, nonfatal crashes were not included in the analysis.

Interventions to the Infrastructure

The evidence-based literature review question asked "What is the evidence for the effect of modifications of the infrastructure of the physical environment (e.g., roadways, signage, lighting) on the driving ability, performance, and safety of the older adult?" As mentioned previously, information prior to 1999 was taken from the *Highway Design Handbook: For Older Drivers and Pedestrians* (Staplin et al., 2001), because this document provides guidelines for the highway design for communities across the United States. Although this report is exhaustive, it is not based on an evidence-based review of the literature; however, it does represent the current status of the science in the engineering and human factors industry prior to 1999 (see Appendix D for a comprehensive summary of this report). The studies examined in the review since 1999 focusing on intervention to the infrastructure included four studies that investigated signage specific to color, reflectiveness, location, fonts, and familiar versus unfamiliar signs. The evidence supports specific colors and fonts, yet all of the studies lacked applicability to real-life driving environments, because they were conducted either on computers or airport runways.

Chrysler, Carlson, and Hawkins (2002) examined the effects of sign color and retro reflective sheeting on the nighttime legibility of three fonts commonly used for highway signage. This Level I randomized mixed-factor design study was conducted on the runways of an abandoned Air Force base. Although there were significant legibility benefits from using orange signs with Type VII or Type IX coatings, there is some question regarding how much of a safety benefit can be expected from the relatively small improvements in legibility distance. In addition, the authors reported that older drivers performed more poorly when reading the orange signs typically used in construction zones.

Ho, Scialfa, Caird, and Graw (2001) examined the effects of age, clutter, and lighting on locating traffic signs in a Level I randomized mixed-factor design study. Older adults were slower and less accurate in locating the traffic signs. This study was limited because it consisted of static images on a computer screen, which is not representative of the driving experience.

The nighttime legibility distance of the Clearview alphabet was evaluated by Carlson (2001) in a Level I mixed-factor study conducted in an abandoned Air Force base. The results of the study indicated that the Clearview font performed significantly better than the Series E (Modified) font, particularly for older drivers. Although Carlson's findings were significant, the effects noted may not be meaningful in real-world applications because the Clearview font may provide only marginal increases in available reading time and legibility distance.

Kline, Buck, Sell, Bolan, and Dewar (1999) conducted a Level I study and found that legibility thresholds were lower for older versus younger participants and for familiar (standard) signs versus unfamiliar signs and that older drivers use an age-related compensatory ability to acquire sign messages. The results of this Level I randomized mixed-factor study would need to be repeated in a field study before definitive conclusions could be made, because the optical-blurring technique used in the laboratory did not physically change the distance between the observer and the sign as would be seen when driving in the real world.

Carmeli, Coleman, Omar, and Brown-Cross (2000) conducted a Level I randomized mixed-factor study to determine the effect of environmental conditions on walking speed in elderly people able to ambulate independently. Exclusion criteria for the study included a history of stroke, myocardial infarction, and inflammatory arthritis. Participants were randomized to two indoor and outdoor trials. In both contexts, participants navigated crosswalk at preferred place and as quickly as possible. Although both were simulated environments, the indoor trial was a tiled, level walkway, while the outdoor crosswalk was designed to meet the specification of an average flat residential crosswalk. The results indicated that participants walked more slowly outdoors than indoors and were less able to increase their "quickly-as-possible" pace during the outdoor trial. The authors indicated that environmental factors such as uneven terrain and variability in light, wind, humidity, and temperature may have contributed to the results. A limitation of the study is that the number of exclusion criteria may make it difficult to generalize the results to the overall older adult population.

Interventions to the Automobile

The evidence-based literature review question asked "What is the evidence for the effect of automobile-related modifications on the driving ability, performance, and safety of the older adult?"

The studies examined in the review on modifications to the automobile included 3 studies that investigated window tinting, 1 that looked at effect of veiling glare on windshield from the dashboard, one study that examined the location of vehicle controls and displays, and 1 study that examined an adapted cruise-control system. The evidence reveals that darker tinting in vehicles is detrimental to visibility for older drivers. The studies reviewed support the need for simplified placement of vehicle controls and displays while supporting automated systems such as adapted cruise control.

Freedman, Zador, and Staplin (1993) examined how tinted rear windows affected driving during simulation for older and younger drivers. The use of deeply tinted windows is of concern because they transmit less light than less deeply tinted glass and therefore reduce driver visibility. In this Level I randomized mixed-factor study, each participant viewed five common roadway objects at various contrast levels, which were projected onto screens located to the rear of a simulated vehicle, as the driver looked through four transmittance levels of tinted windows. Performance decreased for older drivers and on trials in which there was decreased transmittance (more deeply tinted glass) and contrast. Older drivers were less likely to detect objects than younger drivers. The authors concluded that safety of backing maneuvers was significantly reduced for both groups in cars with rear window tinting that decreases rear window transmittance to a level of 53% or less. According to the authors, older adults may have an increased risk of not detecting low-contrast objects with reduced-transmittance windows below 70%.

LaMotte, Ridder, Yeung, and De Land (2000) studied how different levels of window tinting affects driving performance in a Level II nonrandomized mixed-factor design. For older drivers in a simulated driving situation, a tint of 57% significantly reduced middle to high spatial frequency contrast sensitivity. The study demonstrated that dark tints (18% transmittance) had detrimental effects on the driver's vision, regardless of age. This study was limited by a lack of randomization of the treatment.

The effect of tinting car front-side windows was studied by Burns, Nettlebeck, White, and Wilson (1999) in a Level I randomized mixed-factor design study. The results of the study indicate that a reduction of visible light transmittance resulted in decreased driving performance for older adults, except in some optimal driving conditions.

Schumann, Flannagan, Sivak, and Traube (1997) studied veiling glare conditions, which occur when reflected images from the top of the dashboard are superimposed on the image of the road scene in the windshield. These images can impair visual performance by reducing the contrast of objects in the road scene. Two groups (elderly people and young adults) performed a detection task of a pedestrian during veiling glare conditions. The results indicated that both the angle at which the windshield is mounted (windshield rake angle) and dashboard reflectance have measurable effects on visual performance, and effects were particularly pronounced when a large rake angle was combined with high dashboard reflectance. This study implies that decreased contrast sensitivity is an important factor to consider in determining the type of car that best meets the needs of an elderly client. However, other factors that may have some influence on veiling glare, such as dashboard gloss and texture, were not included in the analysis of this Level I study.

Laux (1991) conducted a Level I randomized mixed-factor design study that examined whether age was a factor in how drivers located controls and display systems when driving in unfamiliar vehicles. Older drivers took a significantly longer time to locate controls they might need regularly as well as those that would be needed infrequently.

Adapted cruise control (ACC) adjusts the speed of a car in response to the speed set by the driver and measurements of the distance to the vehicle ahead (Fancher et al., 1998). In a Level III before-and-after study, 108 older drivers and younger drivers drove a test vehicle with ACC for either a 2-week or 5-week period. After an orientation session, drivers could choose when and how to use the system. Features of the ACC system included a "sweep" sensor that detected distance and rate of closure to the vehicle ahead and a "cut-in" sensor that detected when other vehicles cut in front of the driver. The ACC system did not operate at less than 35 mph (56 km/hr); during system failure; or during reduced visibility conditions, such as salt spray, snow, and fog. The results indicated that drivers used the system 20% to 100% of the time when conditions were favorable. Although older drivers used the ACC more than younger drivers, both groups used ACC most frequently for speeds over 55 mph (88.5 km/hr). In general, older drivers set the system to allow for more space between cars than younger drivers, and ACC usage by the older drivers was greater at the beginning than the end of the study. Ninety-five percent of the older drivers favored the use of ACC and stated that they would use the system in the future. The study was limited by the lack of a control group.

Implications of the Evidence-Based Literature Review

The results from the studies reported in the evidence-based literature review support the theory behind the Haddon matrix, which suggests that multiple factors contribute to older driver crashes, injuries, and fatalities. The literature suggests that individually, and in combination with each other, the person, the social environment, the physical environment, and the car all contribute to older drivers' crashes. As a result of the multifaceted influence on older driver safety, interventions to support older adult performance and safety in driving target each of the factors contributing to crashes.

Interventions aimed at the person addressed the impact of educational programs, considered the role of passengers, and examined remediation for vision and cognitive and motor deficits associated with aging and stroke on driving performance and safety. The research supports the need for occupational therapy practitioners to consider multiple avenues of intervention rather than solely considering adaptive equipment to support driving performance. Based on individual needs, interventions conducted with drivers should incorporate programs addressing impaired vision, cognition and motor skills, pharmaceutical treatments, technology, and educational programs.

From a population-based perspective, occupational therapy practitioners have a role to educate policymakers about limitations in screening tools, the impact of aging and illness on driving performance, and the impact of driving cessation. The literature review identified successful mechanisms to reduce fatalities through driving restrictions and increased relicensing requirements. Although more stringent relicensing policies can reduce automobile-related fatalities, the literature also demonstrated increases in pedestrian and bicycle fatalities when relicensure is so strict that there is a high prevalence of license forfeiture.

More effective evaluation programs and rigorous licensure policies increase the need for transportation alternatives to allow older adults to remain mobile throughout the community. The literature suggests that older adults are not entirely comfortable with using many of the transit services currently available. There is evidence that programs such as the Independent Transportation Network can support community mobility, sustain business clientele, and maintain fiscal viability.

The literature described how design and modifications to the infrastructure to intersection design,

signage, roadway markings, lighting, and construction supports older driver performance. Specific features, such as traffic signals allowing protected left turns, larger signs in Clearview font, roundabouts, and luminescent high-contrast roadway markings, foster enhanced negotiation of roadways by older adults.

Another area of intervention addressing the needs of the older adult population rather than the individual driver is design or modifications to the vehicles. The literature reviewed discussed the effects of window tinting, water-resistant window and mirror treatments, instrument panel displays, and angle of the windshield with resultant dashboard reflection. The research revealed that deeper window tinting had a detrimental effect on participants' ability to visually decipher the driving environment. The evidence suggests that water-resistant treatment on windows does not improve driving performance. Older adults' visibility within the vehicle was hampered with unfamiliar vehicle control/display location and smaller characters. Visibility also is improved with smaller windshield rake angles and low dashboard reflectance.

In general, the evidence-based literature review identifies numerous strategies to improve or maintain driving ability in general and for older drivers in particular. The community mobility literature is less conclusive in addressing the question of participation by older adults. Innovative transportation programs and research to determine the program's effectiveness and sustainability are in the early stages of development. Additional research is necessary to ascertain the occupational performance outcomes of community mobility programs.

Strengths and Limitations of Studies

The evidence-based literature review yielded many high-quality studies. Of the 56 studies included in the review, nearly half (26) of the articles reviewed were at the highest level of evidence (Level I), and 22 of the articles were at the second highest level of evidence (Level II). Many of the studies were population based, and thus the results can be generalized. The review was also inclusive in that it included literature and reports from different health-related disciplines as well as engineers and incorporated international literature.

Several limitations of the review and of the individual studies need to be kept in mind. The review was extremely broad and included a wide range of interventions due to the foundation in the Haddon matrix and subsequent inclusion of the person, the social environment, the physical environment, and the car. In addition to a vast array of interventions, the studies varied between the well population and people with disabilities. Although the diversity of disciplines in which the studies were conducted offers a broad perspective, only 3 of the studies came from the occupational therapy literature. The limited representation from the occupational therapy literature hinders the direct applicability of the results to occupational therapy practice. Several population-based studies used the Fatal Accident Reporting System database as the outcome variable. Although this is a widely used, well-respected national database, it includes only fatalities and does not include all traffic incidents.

Other studies used state crash databases that have inclusion criteria such as a tow-away or $1,500 worth of damage. Many traffic incidents not meeting the inclusion criteria, or smaller incidents, such as parking lot crashes, personal property damage, or running over curbs, are not included in these databases. Studies using traffic violations also have limitations due to nonreported incidents and law enforcement leniency with older adults. The non-population-based studies were limited by small sample sizes. Many of the studies examining interventions to the person had limitations related to lack of control groups, small sample size, and learning effects.

Finally, as reported earlier, the guidelines for highway design for communities across the United States are based on a report published by the U.S. Department of Transportation (Federal Highway Administration, 2001). Although several studies and reports published since 1999 were included, these studies lacked applicability to real-life driving environments because they were conducted either on computers or airport runways.

Clinical Practice, Education, and Research

The various studies included in the literature review used approaches both familiar and not familiar to occupational therapy practitioners and included skills-based interventions, education, modifications to the vehicle, infrastructure design, policy, and community mobility programs. On the basis of the current literature, occupational therapists and occupational therapy assistants should be prepared to provide interventions that are both direct and consultative in nature to meet the multifaceted factors contributing to older driver performance and safety.

The review of the research under discussion reveals that successful interventions share some common features. They include the following:

- Approaches focused on the client's performance skills and on client factors
- Comprehensive licensing programs that consider the impact of aging and illness on performance skills, performance patterns, and client factors
- Community-building efforts for collaborative transportation services that meet the needs of all stakeholders
- Technology to support performance in the IADL of community mobility
- Collaboration with municipal planning entities and roadway engineers to recommend elder-friendly infrastructure that tailors activity demands in consideration of age-related performance skills and client factors and regional performance patterns and contexts
- Consultation with automobile manufacturers specific to elder-friendly vehicle design that consider performance skills and client factors altered by aging and illness, the contexts in which older adults drive, and the performance patterns older adults follow.

Occupational therapy practitioners are uniquely equipped to address the needs of older adults in the area of driving and community mobility based on the professional understanding of the effects of aging and illness on performance; an appreciation for the contribution of driving and community mobility to daily life; and their expertise in task analysis, evaluation, and intervention planning. When evaluating an older adult's ability to drive, occupational therapists consider the client's occupational history and occupational engagement needs while synthesizing information about the client's skills and deficits as well as the context in which the client performs. When planning therapeutic interventions for older adults to support driving and community mobility, occupational therapists should consider the client's need to access services, resources, and other occupations in the community. The client, family, and occupational therapist should work together to develop a plan that best meets community mobility needs while preserving safety. The therapist should assume the roles of consultant, designer, facilitator, advocate, and source of emotional support.

The findings presented in the evidence-based literature review suggest growing opportunities for occupational therapy practice outside of traditional medical settings. There are opportunities for occupational therapists to serve as consultants to medical review boards, community planning boards, transportation safety programs, policy-making groups, aging agencies, transit authorities, and automobile manufacturers. If one views these population-based interventions within the growing public health aspect of occupational therapy practice, the opportunities are plentiful. The case can be made that occupational therapists have an important role not only in helping older adults return to driving when illness or injury has impaired performance but also in the prevention of injury, fatality, and occupational disengagement.

Occupational therapy professional programs are well suited to guide new therapists to address driving and community mobility as an IADL and to describe the specialization of driving rehabilitation and community mobility for the older adult population. At present, students take coursework in psychosocial issues, gerontology, and community-based practice as well as learn concepts related to occupational analysis, assessment, intervention planning, public health, injury prevention, and population-based services. Most educational programs offer content specific to driving rehabilitation, but to varying degrees. Concentrated efforts should be made by all educational programs to include content related to driving rehabilitation as well as a specific focus on older drivers and community mobility. Professional programs can facilitate these learning experiences through cooperative relationships with area clinical programs, guest lecturers, and site visits to driving rehabilitation programs. Overall, educational programs need to foster the recognition of driving and community mobility as an IADL and within the scope of both general and specialized occupational therapy practice.

The implications for occupational therapy research are clear: More well-designed studies addressing the benefits of occupation-based interventions and occupational performance outcomes are needed. Only three of the articles included occupational therapy, but the positive side is that researchers in other disciplines see the value of conducting research related to older drivers, and the results of these studies have application to occupational therapy practice. Although clinical research is typically hampered by its multifaceted nature, it is necessary to provide evidence-based, effective interventions.

There is evidence that interventions to the person, the vehicle, policy, community mobility, and the infrastructure can be effective in supporting driving and community mobility among older adults. Not only does this document serve as a guideline for practice, but it also provides suggestions for occupational therapy research and education.

■ ■ ■

Appendix A.
Preparation and Qualifications of Occupational Therapists and Occupational Therapy Assistants

Who Are Occupational Therapists?

To practice as an occupational therapist, the individual trained in the United States

- Has graduated from an occupational therapy program accredited by the Accreditation Council for Occupational Therapy Education (ACOTE) or predecessor organizations,
- Has successfully completed a period of supervised fieldwork experience required by the recognized educational institution where the applicant met the academic requirements of an educational program for occupational therapists that is accredited by ACOTE or predecessor organizations,
- Has passed a nationally recognized entry-level examination for occupational therapists, and
- Fulfills state requirements for licensure, certification, or registration.

Educational Programs for the Occupational Therapist

These include the following:

- Biological, physical, social, and behavioral sciences
- Basic tenets of occupational therapy
- Occupational therapy theoretical perspectives
- Screening and evaluation
- Formulation and implementation of an intervention plan
- Context of service delivery
- Management of occupational therapy services
- Use of research
- Professional ethics, values, and responsibilities.

The fieldwork component of the program is designed to develop competent, entry-level, generalist occupational therapists by providing experience with a variety of clients across the life span and in a variety of settings. Fieldwork is integral to the program's curriculum design and includes an in-depth experience in delivering occupational therapy services to clients, focusing on the application of purposeful and meaningful occupation and/or research, administration, and management of occupational therapy services. The fieldwork experience is designed to promote clinical reasoning and reflective practice, to transmit the values and beliefs that enable ethical practice, and to develop professionalism and competence in career responsibilities.

Who Are Occupational Therapy Assistants?

To practice as an occupational therapy assistant, the individual trained in the United States

- Has graduated from an associate- or certificate-level occupational therapy assistant program accredited by ACOTE or predecessor organizations,
- Has successfully completed a period of supervised fieldwork experience required by the recognized educational institution where the applicant met the academic requirements of an educational program for occupational therapy assistants that is accredited by ACOTE or predecessor organizations,

- Has passed a nationally recognized entry-level examination for occupational therapy assistants, and
- Fulfills state requirements for licensure, certification, or registration.

Educational Programs for the Occupational Therapy Assistant

These include the following:
- Biological, physical, social, and behavioral sciences
- Basic tenets of occupational therapy
- Screening and assessment
- Intervention and implementation
- Context of service delivery
- Assistance in management of occupational therapy services
- Use of professional literature
- Professional ethics, values, and responsibilities.

The fieldwork component of the program is designed to develop competent, entry-level, generalist occupational therapy assistants by providing experience with a variety of clients across the life span and in a variety of settings. Fieldwork is integral to the program's curriculum design and includes an in-depth experience in delivering occupational therapy services to clients, focusing on the application of purposeful and meaningful occupation. The fieldwork experience is designed to promote clinical reasoning appropriate to the occupational therapy assistant role, to transmit the values and beliefs that enable ethical practice, and to develop professionalism and competence in career responsibilities.

Regulation of Occupational Therapy Practice

All occupational therapists and occupational therapy assistants must practice under federal and state law. Currently, 50 states, the District of Columbia, Puerto Rico, and Guam have enacted laws regulating the practice of occupational therapy.

Note. The majority of this information is taken from the *Standards for an Accredited Educational Program for the Occupational Therapist* (AOTA, 1999a), *Standards for an Accredited Educational Program for the Occupational Therapy Assistant* (AOTA, 1999b), and *Standards of Practice* (AOTA, 2005a).

■ ■ ■

Appendix B.
Adaptive Equipment

The following describes some of the basic adaptive equipment used in driving and community mobility along with special considerations for some of the equipment. The information below does not represent an inclusive list of all the possible equipment used in driving rehabilitation and community mobility. Occupational therapy practitioners wishing to advance their knowledge and expertise in adaptive equipment should participate in continuing education activities and work directly with an adaptive equipment dealer.

Steering Devices

Clients who have use of only one arm can benefit from an adaptive steering device that allows them to move the steering wheel through a complete rotation without releasing or changing grip. Whether due to impairment of one arm or occupation of the arm by a hand control, the ball-bearing mechanism in steering devices allows for single-arm operation of the steering wheel. The location of installation must consider the client's ability to reach and maintain a comfortable upper-extremity position during straight driving but should also consider obstruction of the airbag on deployment. Since the development of airbags mounted in the center of steering wheels, the ideal driver hand position is at the 4 o'clock and 8 o'clock positions. This grip position is recommended for all drivers so that the forearms do not cross the center of the steering wheel and cannot cause injury to the upper extremities or face on airbag deployment. When possible, steering devices should be installed in the lower quadrants of the steering wheel to reduce the amount of time the driver's arm crosses over the airbag.

The most commonly used steering device is a spinner knob, which includes a base firmly attached to the steering wheel and a removable knob that inserts into the ball-bearing mechanism. The spinner knob, which is shaped like a small doorknob, requires the client to

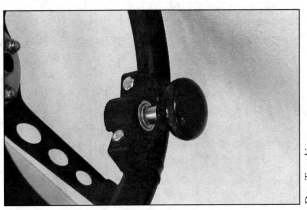

Spinner knob

have full control of the hand used for steering, allowing for sustained grasp.

Individuals with less strength or control in the steering hand with control in the wrist need a device that provides more support to the hand and can be managed more passively. For single-hand steering in these cases, clients may have more control using a palm spinner, which looks like a universal cuff, which maintains the forearm in a prone position.

For drivers with little to no control in the hand, such as clients with quadriplegia, a steering device that holds the hand more firmly is required. In these

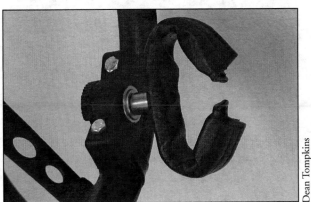

Palm spinner

cases, a tri pin is the best option. The tri pin is configured with three equal-length posts attached to a base that fits into the steering device base on the steering wheel. The posts sit perpendicular to the plane of the steering wheel. The fingers are flexed around the top pin while the other two pins support the hand and wrist maintaining the hand in the device. Some drivers prefer a modified version that consists of a single post rather than three, allowing for a neutral forearm while driving.

Clients with upper-extremity amputations require a different steering device that provides a surface to grasp. The amputee ring consists of a rotating ring into which drivers can insert a prosthesis hook and steer with complete control.

Accelerating and Braking Devices

Clients may have difficulty using the factory-installed vehicle equipment to operate the accelerator and brake. Lack of motor control, absence of sensation, decreased strength or range of motion, loss of a limb, abnormal muscle tone, or short leg length in the right lower extremity may all lead to a need for acceleration or braking devices.

Deficits isolated to the right leg that leave the left leg intact call for installation and training with a left-foot accelerator, which consists of an alternate accelerator pedal that is positioned to the left of the manufacturer-installed brake with a horizontal bar at the base

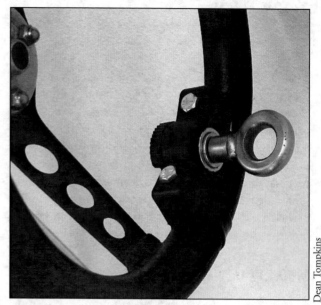
Amputee ring

extending toward the manufacturer-installed accelerator. An additional component to the left-foot accelerator is a vertical bar extending upward from the horizontal bar that depresses the manufacturer-installed accelerator when the driver operates the left-foot accelerator. Some left-foot accelerators come with a block to prohibit accidental operation of the manufacturer-installed accelerator with the resting right foot. Clients

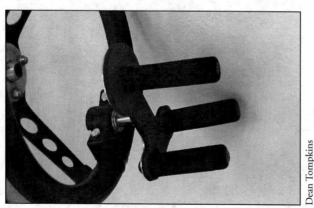
Tri pin

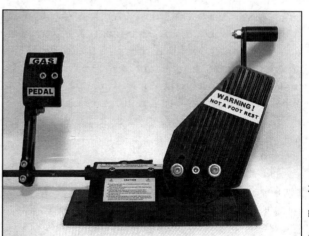
Left-foot accelerator

must then learn to use the left foot for all acceleration and braking control of the vehicle. Although this is typically an easy transition to make for most drivers, cognitive impairments often slow the learning process because of the opposite nature of this movement compared with previously learned patterns.

There is debate in the field about the safety of the left-foot accelerator related to the ability to use the left leg in an automatic manner. An accepted position on the use of the left-foot accelerator is that the low cost and ease of installation should not override considerations of client safety and competent operation.

Individuals with short lower extremities may not be able to use factory-installed pedals for gas and brake operation. By providing the necessary reach, pedal extenders can serve as a low-tech solution that allows the person to drive using typical patterns. For individuals who are short but not of short stature, a recommendation can be made to purchase a vehicle with power pedal extenders that offer a telescoping option on the manufacturer-installed brake and accelerator pedals.

Some drivers have deficits affecting both lower extremities, making it impossible to use the factory-installed brake and accelerator and eliminating a left foot accelerator as an option. In these instances, an alternate method of depressing the accelerator and brake must be provided. One of the options is hand controls, which are available in a variety of motion-related models. Many hand controls can include installation of horn and high-beam switches so that the person can operate these secondary controls without releasing the accelerator or brake. Hand controls are usually installed on the left side of the steering column for ease of operation with maximal space for operation without hitting a center console.

Push–pull hand controls require that the driver push the control forward, toward the front of the vehicle, to brake and pull back in the opposite direction to accelerate. Good hand control is necessary to use this equipment. This control is relatively easy to operate, as it offers two distinct movements for acceleration and braking, thus minimizing confusion.

The push-right angle control requires a push-forward motion for braking and a downward motion at a right angle to the braking motion for acceleration. Push-right angle hand controls offer an option similar to the push–pull control, but less space inside the vehicle is required for operation. In addition, the push-right angle control does not require full control of the hand and provides a less fatiguing position during prolonged acceleration. An additional and control option is the push-twist, which uses a similar pushing forward for braking but a forward twist, similar to a motorcycle accelerator that is used to apply gas. The choice of hand controls is individual and depends on several factors, including the client's hand use, the size of the client's legs, the size of the vehicle interior, and the client's ability to learn the required movements for operation.

Hand controls can be installed to provide clients with quadriplegia the proper position and angle for operation to accommodate for wheelchair seating and decreased strength and range of motion. These controls are mounted to the floor of a van, creating a different fulcrum of movement than is used with other hand controls. A tri pin handle is typically used with these hand controls to allow for a secure hold by the driver's hand.

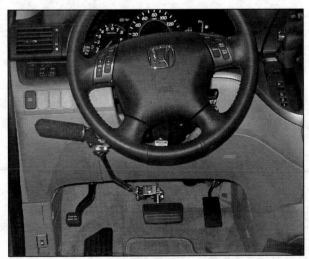

Hand controls

Dean Tompkins

If a client's left hand is operating a hand control, and the right hand is managing all steering, then the act of releasing the accelerator or the steering wheel to use the directional signal becomes difficult. If necessary, a crossover turn signal can be installed so the right hand can operate the signal from the position of the steering device. This illustration shows the crossover turn signal crossing under the steering column, but it is often installed in a position that is crosses over the steering column.

Other Equipment

The previous examples of adaptive equipment do not represent an all-inclusive list of available products. They do, however, represent the most commonly used devices that can meet the needs of most clients. Other types of equipment include an assortment of convex mirrors to compensate for decreased neck rotation or limited visual field; an array of wheelchair/scooter lifts for use in cars and vans; any combination of lowered floor/raised roof/lifts/ramps to allow wheelchair-dependent individuals access to their vans; and high-technology equipment for computerized steering, acceleration, and braking and push-button ignition. Before making decisions about which equipment

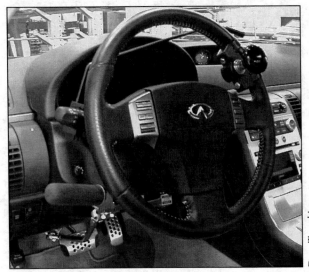

Dean Tompkins

Crossover turn signal

would best meet the needs of specific diagnoses, the therapist can visit a local adaptive equipment vendor to view and manipulate each type of equipment. A complete activity analysis with each piece of equipment should be completed so that the occupational therapist understands the amount of range of motion and extent of strength required for effective operation.

Clients who have difficulty isolating or manipulating keys or operating the ignition of a vehicle because of fine motor coordination deficits may benefit from adaptive key chains. Adaptive key chains come in a variety of styles to foster independence by firmly holding a single key isolated. Another function of adaptive key chains is providing a larger surface for turning with great leverage or allowing for gross movement to rotate the key.

Convex mirrors provide for greater visual access to the driving environment for drivers with decreased neck or trunk rotation, limited lateral eye gaze, or vestibular problems with head-turning. These curved mirrors contain more of the driving environment to compensate for the driver's inability to look directly. Like adaptive key chains, convex mirrors come in a variety of styles, some of which replace or add on to the manufacturer's rearview mirror; some which are placed on the side-view mirrors with adhesive; and some, for clients with significantly restricted neck mobility, that can be attached to the hood of the vehicle.

Some clients may be able to operate a vehicle easily but have difficulty entering or exiting their vehicles. For these individuals, assistive seating may be the best option. Assistive seating options range from low-tech swivel platforms placed on the driver's seat to high-tech automated seats that replace the manufacturer's driver's seat and rotate the driver 90 degrees and help him or her transfer from sitting to standing.

Although most of the adaptive equipment used in vehicles improves occupational performance and allows drivers to be independent, there are negative implications of using these devices. All adaptive equipment is considered an aftermarket product and was not included in any testing to measure the crashworthiness of vehicles. Additional equipment can prove to be hazardous in the event of an automobile crash or can even obstruct the operation of vehicle safety features, such as airbags. Most clients are eager to have equipment to restore their independence, but all clients should be informed consumers. Occupational therapy practitioners should consider the implications of the prescribed aftermarket products and educate clients accordingly so that clients can make their own decisions about balancing independence and injury prevention.

Transit Equipment

Clients using transportation alternatives require special modification considerations for accessing transit, entering and exiting, and using the services. In addition to modifications to the environment, therapists should work with transit agencies to provide sensitivity training to drivers, schedulers, and other staff who have contact with consumers. It is especially important that drivers receive training to ensure that they are sensitive to the needs of passengers with disabilities. Such training must include the mechanics of how to board and secure persons who are in wheelchairs. Driver training should always emphasize safe driving. In addition, agencies that provide travel training or travel companions can be helpful in orienting clients to a new service.

Before considering the accessiblity of a bus, van, or train, therapists must consider how easily the client can get to the service. The path to the pickup and drop-off points should be clear and wide enough to accommodate a wheelchair or walker. Bus stops and shelters should be sized adequately to allow wheelchair users to wait safely and under cover if possible.

Entrance to and exiting the transportation vehicle is of next concern. The Americans with Disabilities Act (ADA) Title II states that transit agencies must comply with accessibility laws when purchasing new vehicles and make good-faith efforts to purchase accessible used buses. This legislation also requires that transit agencies provide paratransit services for individuals who are unable to use public system. To meet the needs of

individuals with disabilities, all transit agencies have at least some buses with accessible entrances.

The most common adaptations to buses are low-floor buses or kneeling buses. Many low-floor buses can board wheelchair users directly from a raised sidewalk, whereas a kneeling bus lowers the floor at the entrance for easy entry. Some buses use systems that include a foldout ramp or a use a sliding ramp under the floor. In addition to floor changes, many buses have grab bars or handles for travelers to use to assist with balance and mobility needs. Regardless of the system of entry, the purpose is to allow people and child strollers to enter and exit the bus without needing to ascend high steps.

Access to trains and subways by persons with disabilities is another important part of accessible public transportation. Access to train or subway platforms varies among stations or among different cities. Many subway stations are far below ground and require elevators to bring travelers with disabilities to the platform level. Therapists should understand the system used by the transit agencies to identify which stations are accessible by elevator to facilitate client education. Access to trains is easier to accommodate than access to buses, because there are fewer train stations, they are usually farther apart than bus stops, and wheelchair access is necessary on only one car per train. Additionally, the raised platform of train stations typically provides a level entrance for all passengers. Because the entrance to the train or subway is level, it should be clearly marked with a warning strip with a different color, texture, or lighting so travelers can see and feel the warning strip under foot or at the touch of a cane used by a blind person. To meet the needs of persons with disabilities, the car doors need to be wide enough to accommodate wheelchairs, walkers, and other mobility devices. The space inside the cars should be designed such that a wheelchair can be parked or the uses transferred into a regular seat.

Once clients are inside the transit vehicle, there must be a mechanism to secure wheelchairs to eliminate shifting and prevent injury to the client and other transit users. Depending on the system used in the individual transit vehicle, travelers in wheelchairs are secured facing forward or sideways. The mechanism to secure the wheelchair is typically a wheel clamp or belt that attaches to the frame of the chair. In addition to securing the chair, the passenger is secured with a standard seat belt. Clients and caregivers should be taught about these wheelchair securement systems and learn to advocate for the use of the systems when riding as passengers.

The best transportation alternative for some clients may be the existing transit system, whereas others may benefit from smaller vehicles for door-to-door service and nonfixed route services. Private transportation agencies or paratransit divisions of large transit agencies typically use smaller vehicles such as vans, small buses, or taxis. Many of these vehicles need to be equipped with modifications to accommodate wheelchairs, so lifts and ramps are installed in the vans and small buses. These services operate either on a door-to-door system, which requires individuals to plan ahead and schedule the service and pickup times. Service routes usually follow a semifixed route designed to pass near the homes of seniors and persons with disabilities as well as major trip destinations such as shopping areas, schools, and rehabilitation centers. The routes are semifixed to allow drivers to deviate a short distance from a fixed route to pick up a person who has telephoned for service from home. In some cases, these smaller vehicle services are used to transport individuals from their homes to accessible bus routes or railroad stations.

Travelers who use transit services must be able to receive information about the service with regard to schedules, routes, hours of operation, and the next stop. The modification of signage and information is critical to ensure that all passengers are aware of their surroundings and travels. Information should be provided in visual, tactile, and audible formats. This information should be accessible both throughout the transit station and in the vehicle. Audible announcements need to be understandable and provided at a volume that does not interfere with other audible cues.

■ ■ ■

Appendix C.
Evidence Table

Evidence Table

Author/Year	Study Objectives	Level/Design/Participants	Intervention & Outcome Measures	Results	Limitations
Allen et al. (1991)	Establish the effectiveness of a navigation system in early prompting to drivers for taking an alternate route for avoiding traffic congestions	II—Mixed-factor, nonrandomized control trial Five groups: 4 intervention and 1 control N = 277 Older drivers were included in study, but the number was not reported.	Intervention groups: 1 of 4 navigation systems (static navigation system, dynamic map system, advanced map system, or route guidance system) Control group Outcomes: ■ Prequestionnaire: Information about participants' background, commuting patterns, and opinions about commuting ■ Postquestionnaire: Past diversion behavior, factors for congestion avoidance, anticipated delay time, and human-factor issues of navigation system ■ Response to traffic congestion scenario	50% of drivers diverted with slowing of traffic with use of navigation system. Middle-age drivers were most likely to divert, and older drivers were least likely to divert. 50% diversion by drivers noted, with delay time reaching 18 min. Diversion was done more frequently during pleasure-related trips than daily commutes.	Weak analytical methodology: low sensitivity and specificity of outcome measures; applicability to real-life situations is limited; no test of significance among groups; number of older drivers participating in the study not reported.

Reference: Allen, R. W., Stein, A. C., Rosenthal, T. J., Ziedman, D., Torres, J. F., & Halati, A. (1991). A human factors study of driver reaction to in-vehicle navigation systems. In *SAE Technical Paper Series* (Paper No. 911680, pp. 83–102). Warrendale, PA: SAE International.

Author/Year	Study Objectives	Level/Design/Participants	Intervention & Outcome Measures	Results	Limitations
Ashman et al. (1994)	Develop and evaluate the efficacy and effectiveness of an intervention to improve safety in older drivers	I—Randomized control trial; 4 groups with different interventions Pre-post measurement N = 105 All participants were older than age 65 and driving on a regular basis.	Group I: Home-based physical therapy to improve posture and upper-limb flexibility (8 weeks) Group II: Home-based perceptual therapy for visual–perception skills (8 weeks) Group III: Driver education program to improving driving skills (1 day for 8 hr) Group IV: Improvement in driving environment Outcome: ■ Drivers Performance Measurement.	Each intervention was reported to be effective in improving driving performance by 7.9% from the baseline performance. No statistical significant difference was reported between groups; however, physical therapy was reported to be most cost-effective compared with the other interventions.	Group IV was tested 3 times, which may have skewed the results.

Reference: Ashman, R. D., Bishu, R. R., Foster, B. G., & McCoy, P. T. (1994). Countermeasures to improve the driving performance of older drivers. *Educational Gerontology, 20*, 567–577.

Study	Objective	Study design/sample	Intervention/method	Results	Comments
Ball et al. (1988)	Describe changes in peripheral visual field and its influence on functional vision and determine effectiveness of training in improving visual skills	I—Randomized control trial Two groups: Intervention I and Intervention II N = 24 (8 participants ages 20–30, 8 participants ages 40–49, and 8 participants age 60–75)	Intervention I: Training using the useful field of view (UFOV) with low distracters. Intervention II: Training using the UFOV with high distracters (5 sessions)	Visual field area was reported to be more affected in older participants compared with younger ones. Improvement in performance noted after practice increased significantly for older participants, resembling that of middle-age participants before practice.	Applicability of the training in improving visual skills for functional activities may be questionable.

Reference: Ball, K. K., Beard, B. L., Roenker, D. L., Miller, R. L., & Griggs, D. S. (1988). Age and visual search: Expanding the useful field of view. *Journal of Optical Society of America, 5,* 2210–2219.

Study	Objective	Study design/sample	Intervention/method	Results	Comments
Burns et al. (1999)	Determine whether road safety is compromised in drivers with tinted front car windows, reducing the visible light transmittance (VLT) to 35%	II—Mixed-factor nonrandomized control trial Experiment I: N = 30; 12 younger and 18 older participants Experiment II: N = 26; 13 younger and 13 older participants	Experiment I: 6 trials for each of the 6 possible combinations of 2 luminance and 3 VLT outcomes: Inspection time in each viewing condition for identification of objects presented Experiment II: 2 levels of luminance (high/low illuminating headlights) and 3 VLT levels (100%, 81.3%, and 35%). Inspection time was similar to Experiment I and recognition of alphanumeric characters.	Experiment I: In optimal driving conditions, the driving performance was not affected by the VLT for the elderly individuals. However, under marginal viewing conditions a VLT of 63% was reported to affect the driving. For young adults, the deterioration in driving was reported with VLT at 20%. Experiment II: Deterioration of driving was consistently related with the decrease in VLT for all elderly individuals and was reported to be significantly deteriorated with VLT level at 35%.	Participants were not randomized to treatment conditions; results of testing in a simulator may not generalize to on-road driving conditions.

Reference: Burns, N. R., Nettlebeck, R., White, M., & Wilson, J. (1999). Effects of car window tinting on visual performance: A comparison of elderly and young drivers. *Ergonomics, 42,* 428–443.

(continued)

Evidence Table *(continued)*

Author/Year	Study Objectives	Level/Design/Participants	Intervention & Outcome Measures	Results	Limitations
Caird et al. (2001)	Determine the effectiveness of the Vision Enhancement System (VES) on the performance of older and younger drivers and identify which aspects in the traffic system (e.g., other vehicles, pedestrians) should be enhanced to improve traffic conditions	I—Randomized control trial Two groups, pretest–posttest N = 48 older adults (ages 67–86) and younger adults (ages 18–32)	Group 1: Conformal visual enhancement system used in different contexts (e.g., baseline, daytime, fog), which is in the form of a blue bar on front and rear bumpers Group 2: Nonconformal VES displays were used during different contexts (e.g., baseline, daytime, fog) while simulated driving tasks were performed. As object approached car, the blue horizontal bar was below the participant's line of sight. Outcomes: ■ Detection time: To identify the pedestrian, decide on an appropriate action, and initiate response ■ Response type when pedestrian appears ■ Lateral separation distance: Distance between participant's vehicle and parked and oncoming vehicle ■ Response in intersection ■ Open-ended questions about VES	While the use of VESs was reported to be more effective during hazardous conditions such as fog, it was not effective during daytime everyday driving. VES was of questionable usefulness for parked and oncoming cars, and highlighting may not be sufficient for a driver to identify an object and react appropriately.	The results reported in the study are not conclusive; therefore, the applicability of the VES in real-world driving in improving safety is limited.

Reference: Caird, J. K., Horrey, W. J., & Edwards, C. J. (2001). *Effects of conformal and nonconformal vision enhancement systems on older-driver performance* (Transportation Research Record No. 1759, Report No. 01-0479, pp. 38–45). Washington, DC: Transportation Research Board.

Author/Year	Study Objectives	Level/Design/Participants	Intervention & Outcome Measures	Results	Limitations
Carlson (2001)	Compare the effectiveness of different microprismatic retroreflective sheetings on legible nighttime distance for reading Clearview signs and alphabets mounted on the roadside	I—Randomized controlled trial, mixed-factor design N = 60 (20 participants ages 18–34, 20 participants ages 35–54, and 20 participants ages 55 and older)	Two cars were used: a 2001 Chevrolet Blazer with halogen headlights and a 1991 Ford Crown Victoria with headlights with a more vertical focus. Signs were positioned either at shoulder height or mounted overhead, in accordance with current signing practices.	For both shoulder-height and overhead-mounted signs, the Clearview signs were significantly more visible than other types. This benefit was more pronounced for older drivers than for younger drivers.	Applicability of the results to real-world driving situations is limited, as the differences between the two types of alphabets and legibility distance is marginal.

	Purpose	Design/Sample	Methods	Results	Comments
			21 test words were placed on the signs, 1 word per sign per trial. Outcomes: ■ Legibility distance to read signs		Strict exclusion criteria for participant selection does not reflect the composition of the older adult population.

Reference: Carlson, P. J. (2001). *Evaluation of Clearview alphabet with microprismatic retroreflective sheetings* (No. FHWA Report FHWA/TX-02/4049-1). Springfield, VA: National Technical Information Service.

	Purpose	Design/Sample	Methods	Results	Comments
Carmeli, Coleman, Omar, & Brown-Cross (2000)	To determine the influence of environment on walking speed in elderly people.	Level I randomized mixed-factors design 13 participants ages 77–88 years (mean age, 83.1 years) from independent-living resident facility. Exclusion criteria included deafness, history of stroke, myocardial infarction, and inflammatory arthritis.	Participants took part in 4 randomly assigned trials, 2 indoors and 2 outdoors. In 1 indoor and 1 outdoor trial, participants were told to cross at preferred pace, while in other trial, participants were told to walk as quickly as possible. Indoor trials were conducted on a level, tiled walkway, and the outdoor trials were on a simulated crosswalk. Outcome: ■ Walking speed.	Participants required more time in outdoor gait trials to walk a standard distance than they did in indoor trials. In addition, participants were less able to increase speed during "as-fast-as-possible" outdoor pace than indoor case. The authors report that these differences may be due to environmental factors such as uneven terrain and variability in lighting, temperature, humidity, and wind.	

Reference: Carmeli, E., Coleman, R., Omar, H. L., & Brown-Cross, D. (2000). Do we allow elderly pedestrians sufficient time to cross the street in safety? *Journal of Aging and Physical Activity, 8,* 51–58.

	Purpose	Design/Sample	Methods	Results	Comments
Chrysler et al. (2002)	Determine effects of font, color, and retroreflective sheeting type on night-time legibility distance	I—Randomized mixed-factor design $N = 24$ Age range: 55–75 years	A Chevrolet 1998 Lumina with low-beam headlights was used. 48 signs were used for identification. 4 sign colors were used: green, orange, white, and yellow. Half were printed with the Highway Series D font. The remaining green signs were printed with Clearview Road Condensed font, and the remaining yellow, orange, and white signs were printed with the D-Modified font. 3 types of retroreflective sheeting were used: Type III, Type VIII, and Type XI. Outcome: ■ Legibility distance for reading signs	A significant difference in terms of color and type of sheeting used was reported: Yellow was the most effective, with a legibility distance of 190 ft (58 m), and orange was worst, with legibility distance of 164 ft (50 m). Type VIII and Type XI ($M = 184$ ft [56 m]) were reported to be the best of all, whereas Type III sheeting ($M = 174$ ft [53 m]) was the worst. Series D font yielded a significantly higher legibility distance (187 ft [57 m]) than the Clearview Condensed font (171 ft [53 m]).	Study is of good quality. The fact that the study was conducted on an Air Force base may limit the generalizability of the results.

Reference: Chrysler, S. T., Carlson, P. J., & Hawkins, H. G. (2002). *Nighttime legibility of ground-mounted signs as a function of font, color, and retroreflective sheeting type* (FHWA Report No. FHWA/TX-03/1796-2). Springfield, VA: National Technical Information Service.

(continued)

Evidence Table (continued)

Author/Year	Study Objectives	Level/Design/Participants	Intervention & Outcome Measures	Results	Limitations
De Waard et al. (1999)	Determine the effectiveness of a driving offense detecting system in improving compliance of drivers with laws and to see whether such a system has any secondary effect on driving behavior	II—Nonrandomized mixed-factor design *N* = 37 (21 participants ages 30–45 and 16 participants ages 60–75)	Intervention was use of the DETER (*Detection, Enforcement*, and *Tutoring for Error Reduction*) system in a driving simulation environment with feedback about traffic violation in both audio and visual forms. 4 trials were conducted, with feedback only during the 2nd and 3rd trials. Outcomes: ■ Effectiveness of system: Changes in driver behavior ■ Driving performance: Control over vehicle's lateral position ■ Rating scale mental effort: To determine mental workload ■ Heart rate and energy expenditure ■ Subjective opinion about the system	Speeding violations were reported to decline significantly for all age groups with feedback from Sessions 1 to 3. With elders this was significantly lower even in the 4th trial. Numbers of stop violation decreased in Trial 3. A difference was observed in the feedback versus no-feedback groups in terms of control over vehicle's lateral position. No difference was detected in mental workload for feedback versus no-feedback groups. No difference in heart rate and energy expenditure was observed for the 2 groups. Acceptance and satisfaction with the system were higher for the older drivers compared with the younger drivers.	A learning effect cannot be ignored in the 4th trial, which might be accountable for improvement in safety in spite of no feedback; reliability of the measurement system was not reported; the outcome was a combined effect of both visual and auditory system. Preference of one system over the other is not conclusive; participants were not randomized to treatment.

Reference: de Waard, D., Hulst, M., & Brookhuis, K. A. (1999). Elderly and young drivers' reaction to an in-car enforcement and tutoring system. *Applied Ergonomics, 30,* 147–157.

Author/Year	Study Objectives	Level/Design/Participants	Intervention & Outcome Measures	Results	Limitations
Dingus, Hulse, et al. (1997)	Investigate effects of age, experience with navigation system, and navigation technique on driving with the Advanced Traveler Information System (ATIS)	II—Nonrandomized mixed-factor design Study 1: *N* = 18 (6 participants ages 16–18, 6 participants ages 35–45, and 6 participants ages 65–73) Study 2: *N* = 12 Study was limited to high-mileage drivers in Orlando, FL.	Studies 1 & 2: 6 navigation configurations were used: (1) turn-by-turn guidance with voice guidance, (2) turn-by-turn guidance without voice guidance, (3) route map with voice guidance, (4) route map without voice guidance, (5) textual paper direction list, and (6) conventional paper map. 4 types of roadway configurations were used: (1) residential streets, (2) 2-lane arterial, (3) multilane arterial, and (4) freeway. Study 3: Naturalistic driving by participants with rental cars	Older drivers consistently showed decreased performance in navigating, eye duration, scanning behavior, and planning and trip times and made significantly more safety-related errors than younger drivers. Results do, however, show that older drivers can substantially benefit from use of ATIS configurations, especially from the route planning and guidance functions of the ATIS. Older drivers benefited more from turn-by-turn information rather	Lack of randomization.

	Purpose	Design	Sample	Outcomes/Methods	Results	Conclusions/Comments
Dingus, Hulse, et al. (1997) (continued)			Study 3: N = 1,203 (220 participants ages 25–35, 431 participants ages 35–44, 319 participants ages 45–54, 130 participants ages 55–64, and 50 participants ages 65 and older)	Outcomes: Studies 1 & 2 ■ Driving performance ■ Navigation performance: Driving safety. Study 3 ■ TravTek: Driver interactions with the vehicle, vehicle location, and speed heading ■ Subjective experience with ATIS	than full route information. Older drivers also did better with redundancy of information (i.e., use of auditory and visual information). Youngest drivers had an easier time learning and using the TravTek, likely because of the computer experience advantages of these users. In the naturalistic study, the majority of drivers used the ATIS when given the choice, but it was unclear whether drivers selected the configuration that was most usable and resulted in the safest driving or were simply not motivated to change from the default condition.	

Reference: Dingus, T. A., Hulse, M. C., Mollenhauer, M. A., Fleischman, R. N., McGhee, D. V., & Manakkal, N. (1997). Effects of age, system experience, and navigation technique on driving with an advanced traveler information system. *Human Factors, 39,* 177–199.

	Purpose	Design	Sample	Outcomes/Methods	Results	Conclusions/Comments
Dingus, McGhee, et al. (1997)	Evaluate the effects of headway maintenance and of collision avoidance warnings (CAS) on driving performance of older and younger drivers	I—Randomized mixed-factor design	Experiment 1: N = 108 (36 participants ages 18–25, 36 participants ages 30–45, and 36 participants ages 65 and older)	Experiment 1: Participants followed a confederate lead vehicle that controlled the braking for the study. 3 visual displays (car, bars, blocks) were presented to alert drivers of dangerous following circumstances. Outcome: ■ Mean and minimum headway. Experiment 2: Participants followed a confederate lead vehicle, and false alarms were interspersed among the CAS signals that indicated the confederate vehicle was actually braking or turning.	Experiment 1: The displays helped participants maintain larger, safer headway distances than without a display. The displays also helped decrease frequency of driving too closely. No differences between age groups were reported. Experiment 2: Younger drivers tended to drive closer to the confederate vehicle but increased the headway between the 2 cars when more false alarms were experienced. Older drivers were more in-sensitive to false alarms; the authors state that this may be due to a tendency to maintain greater distance between cars under all conditions.	Longer-term field studies would be necessary to establish the full effects of false alarms on driver performance.

Reference: Dingus, T. A., McGhee, D. V., Manakkal, N., Jahns, S. K., Carney, C., & Hankey, J. M. (1997). Human factors field evaluations of automotive headway maintenance/collision warning devices. *Human Factors, 39,* 216–229.

(continued)

Evidence Table *(continued)*

Author/Year	Study Objectives	Level/Design/Participants	Intervention & Outcome Measures	Results	Limitations
Eby et al. (2003)	Determine whether the Driving Decisions Workbook increased self-awareness and general knowledge and was perceived as useful for participants and to establish validity of the workbook in identifying driving abilities	III—Before-and-after study *N* = 99 participants ages 65–90 years	Driving Decisions Workbook was used to assess and get feedback from the participants about changes in driving in 37 core areas. Outcomes: ■ Driving Decisions Workbook ■ Road test: A 7-mile (11.3-km) road test with 28 structured maneuvers at specific locations, scored by 3 raters	Awareness about changing driving abilities and physical health was reported by the participants. Additionally, 75% of the participants expressed interest in using the workbook in future. The correlation between the overall workbook score and the overall road-test score of all participants was positively significant. When broken down by category domains for the workbook, responses for both cognition and psychomotor performance were significantly related to driving performance, but only for 64- to 75-year age group.	Both the intervention and the outcomes measurement use the same Driving Decisions Workbook, which might have limited the identification of the true effect; no control group.

Reference: Eby, D. W., Molnar, L. J., Shope, J. T., Vivoda, J. M., & Fordyce, T. A. (2003). Improving older driver knowledge and self-awareness through self-assessment: The driving decisions workbook. *Journal of Safety Research, 34,* 371–381.

Author/Year	Study Objectives	Level/Design/Participants	Intervention & Outcome Measures	Results	Limitations
Fancher et al. (1998)	Test the effectiveness (use and satisfaction) of adapted cruise control (ACC) for older and younger drivers	Level III—pretest–posttest *N* = 108 (36 participants ages 20–30, 36 participants ages 40–50, and 36 participants ages 60–70)	Participants drove a test vehicle for either 2 or 5 weeks. The ACC system installed in the test vehicle included a "sweep" sensor that detected distance and rate of closure to the vehicle ahead and a "cut-in" sensor that detected when other vehicles cut in front of the driver. Outcomes: ■ Driving styles questionnaire ■ Outcome measures included impact of driving task, utilization choice, comfort, and convenience.	Drivers used the system 20%–100% of the time when conditions were favorable. Older drivers used the ACC more than younger drivers, and it was used most frequently for all age groups for speeds over 55 mph (88.5 km/hr). In general, older drivers set the system for longer headways than younger drivers, and ACC usage by older drivers was greater at the beginning than at the end of the study. 95% of older drivers favored the use of ACC and stated that they would use the system in the future.	Lack of control group.

Reference: Fancher, P., Ervin, R., Sayer, J., Hagan, M., Bogard, S., Bareket, Z., et al. (1998). *Intelligent Cruise Control Field Operational Test* (Final Report, Report No. UMTRI-98-17). Ann Arbor: University of Michigan, Transportation Research Institute.

Author	Purpose	Study design and sample	Intervention and outcomes	Results	Limitations
Freedman et al. (1993)	Investigate effects of low transmittance of rear window on low/medium contrast visibility in a passenger car	I—Randomized mixed-factor design N = 48 (24 participants ages 18–55, 12 participants ages 56–74, and 12 participants ages 75–90)	4 transmittance levels and 5 road-side objects with different levels of contrast were projected onto the rear- and side-view mirrors of a simulated vehicle. Outcomes: ■ Measure of target detection: Location identification of the target ■ Object detection: Both location and identification of the object presented ■ Response time in identification	Performance generally decreased with increasing age and with decreasing transmittance and contrast. Safety of backing maneuvers may be significantly reduced for all drivers in cars with tinting that decrease rear window transmittance to a level of 53% or less. Older adults may have an increase in risk of not detecting low-contrast objects with reduced transmittance windows below 70%.	Use of simulator may make it difficult to generalize to on-road conditions and may underestimate errors of detection. Age-related deficits may have been underestimated for detection due to this sample having a higher level of low-contrast sensitivity than a more randomly sampled broader population.

Reference: Freedman, M., Zador, P., & Staplin, L. (1993). Effects of reduced transmittance film on automobile rear window visibility. *Human Factors, 35,* 535–550.

Author	Purpose	Study design and sample	Intervention and outcomes	Results	Limitations
Freund (2002)	Develop and test innovative transportation programs within an independent transportation network that was designed to meet the community mobility needs of older adults	II—Nonrandomized control trial Sample comprised older persons in Portland, ME, using the independent transportation network; because this was community based, number of potential participants was not known.	Intervention: Ride-and-shop program. Older adults or family members were able to pay for transportation services, and retail merchants contributed to the financial support of the service. Control: No intervention	Rides to participating merchants were greater in the experimental group. A follow-up survey reported overall satisfaction with the program by merchants as well as the older adult study participants.	Lack of randomization; lack of cost–benefit analysis. Increase in use of services by intervention group may be due to increased attention paid by family members sponsoring rides. Numbers of older individuals who participated in the project not reported.

References: Freund, K. (2002). *Pilot testing innovative payment operations for independent transportation for the elderly.* (Transit-IDEA Project 18 Final Report.) Washington, DC: Transportation Research Board.

Author	Purpose	Study design and sample	Intervention and outcomes	Results	Limitations
Gish et al. (1999)	Investigate the efficacy of a Vision Enhancement System (VES) as a countermeasure for preventing night driving crashes and to determine whether there is a relationship between risk perceived by a driver and driving speed	II—Nonrandomized mixed-factor design N = 8 (4 participants ages 26–36 and 4 participants ages 56–70)	Two groups: (1) VES present and (2) VES absent. Each group was presented with 32 trials, which were combinations of different factors, such as age, glare, location, task, and target. Outcome: ■ Distance for detecting target: Target onset distance	Detection of the target was higher with the use of VES than with no use of VES only for glare condition and target location. The younger drivers were more enthusiastic about the usefulness of the display and generally more willing to use it, whereas the older drivers were more cautious and less positive about the benefits of the display.	Small sample size; not randomized. Study was conducted on an abandoned Air Force base, so it may be difficult to generalize the results to on-road conditions. Period of VES use may have been too short to be accepted by older adults.

Reference: Gish, K. W., Staplin, L., & Perel, M. (1999). Human factors issues related to use of vision enhancement systems. In *Research on intelligent transportation systems, human factors, and advanced traveler information system design and effects* (Transportation Research Record 1694). Washington, DC: Transportation Research Board.

(continued)

Evidence Table (continued)

Author/Year	Study Objectives	Level/Design/Participants	Intervention & Outcome Measures	Results	Limitations
Grabowski et al. (2004)	Describe whether state driver licensing renewal policies are associated with fatality rates among older drivers	II—Retrospective cohort study/observational cohort study N = 74,428 older adults ages 65 and older and 231,488 control participants ages 25–64	The authors examined license renewal policies of different states (e.g., in-person renewal, vision test, road test), controlling for factors such as speed limits, use of seat belts, and intoxication level. Outcome: ■ Use of the Fatality Analysis Reporting System in determining number of fatalities within 30 days of crash	States with an in-person license renewal policy had lower fatality rates for drivers ages 85 and older (incident ratio rate of 0.83). States with vision assessments prior to renewal had lower fatality rates for drivers ages 65–74. Road tests and varying length of renewal periods were not associated with numbers of fatalities.	The Fatality Analysis Reporting System omits fatalities occurring more than 30 days after a crash. Variables omitted by the study as control variables (e.g., driving conditions, other traffic regulations) could have an impact on the number of crashes.

Reference: Grabowski, D. C., Campbell, C. M. & Morrissey, M. A. (2004). Elderly licensure laws and motor vehicle fatalities. *Journal of the American Medical Association, 291,* 2840–2846.

Author/Year	Study Objectives	Level/Design/Participants	Intervention & Outcome Measures	Results	Limitations
Guerrier & Fu (2002), Test 1	Evaluate the effectiveness of different traffic control devices for older drivers	III—Pretest–posttest N = 51 participants over ages 55 and older	All participants drove during the daytime on a fixed route in Miami, FL. Participants took cognitive assessments, visual assessments, and visual acuity tests before taking part in the study. Outcomes: ■ Drivers named traffic control devices and described visibility of lane markings to a researcher who was in the back seat of car. ■ Preferences of traffic control devices	Larger text on overhead and advance street signs could be read from a greater distance than smaller text, and the authors recommend the use of 12-in. (30.5-cm) lettering. Six-in. (15-cm) lane markings were generally more visible than 4-in. (10-cm) lane markings. The authors report the need to maintain upkeep of markers, as there was difficulty identifying worn lane markings in some conditions. There was no difference in preference of participants for traditional or offset left-turn lanes.	Lack of randomization; recall bias, because participants were asked to compare current lane markings to those previously encountered, and time delays between markings were not reported. Insufficient information regarding features of intersections.
Guerrier & Fu (2002), Test 2A	Evaluate the legibility distance for identifying street names with the use of the Clearview, Highway C, and Highway D fonts	I—Randomized mixed-factor design N = 37 participants ages 65 and older	Ground-mounted signs: Two signs using only Highway C and Clearview 6-in. (15-cm) fonts. These signs were placed on the medians of 4-lane arterials with a speed limit of 30 mph (48 km/hr).	Ground-mounted signs: Even though the Clearview font had a larger mean legibility distance (110 ft [33.5 m]) than Highway C and D, the difference was significant only for Highway C.	The use of high-beam lights limits the generalizability to on-road daytime driving.

			Advance signs: 3 signs using the Clearview, Highway C, and Highway D 8-in. (20-cm) fonts. These signs were placed on the side of 2-lane roadways with a speed limit of 30 mph (48 km/hr). All drivers used high-beam lights in after-sunset driving conditions. Outcome: ■ Legibility distance for reading the signs: Measured as distance between the vehicle and signs	Advance signs: There was no significant difference between the Clearview and Highway C fonts. Divided-attention skill of the participants was a significant predictor of distance for reading road signs. Age was not a significant predictor for being able to read signs.	Varying ambient light: The authors report the presence of different ambient light conditions during driving testing, which might had some effects on reading distances.
Guerrier & Fu (2002), Test 2A *(continued)*					
Guerrier & Fu (2002), Test 2B	Evaluate the visibility of different lane marking treatments for older drivers	III—Pretest-posttest *N* = 22 participants ages 65 and over	Participants were passengers in a car on the Florida Turnpike. Different marking tapes were applied to half-mile sections of the turnpike. Participants took cognitive assessments, visual assessments, and visual acuity tests before taking part in the study. Outcomes: ■ Participants reported directional shifts of road (left, right, straight ahead) ■ Rating of overall and relative visibilities of lane markers	There were no significant differences between any of the treatments tested.	Lack of randomization; test was conducted under a limited set of roadway conditions (clear and dry), and thus the results may not be generalizable to other road conditions.

Reference: Guerrier, J. H., & Fu, S. H. (2002). *Elder Roadway User Program test sections and effectiveness study—Final report* (Contract No. BB-901, University of Miami Project No. 669535). [Available from Florida Department of Transportation Research Center, 605 Suwannee Street, N.S. 30, Tallahassee, FL 32399-0450]

(continued)

Evidence Table (continued)

Author/Year	Study Objectives	Level/Design/Participants	Intervention & Outcome Measures	Results	Limitations
Hakamies-Blomqvist et al. (1996)	Evaluate and compare the effects of age-based medical screening on improving safety and reducing fatalities for drivers in Finland and Sweden	II—Nonrandomized cohort design Participants were all licensed drivers born before 1960.	No intervention; however, the comparison was made in terms of impact of age-related driving license renewal laws between Sweden and Finland. In Sweden, there is no age-related medical screening or review, and license renewal is not required. In Finland, after age 45, individuals need to pass medical and vision examinations every 5 years to keep their licenses active. After age 70, a medical review by a physician is needed, and renewal time gets shorter. Outcomes: ■ Licensure rate ■ Accident and fatality rate for drivers ■ Fatalities for moped riders, cyclists, and pedestrians	Licensure rates for those older than age 70 was 44.2 in Sweden and 14.6 in Finland. Accident and fatality rates for drivers were similar in both countries, but there was a significant increase in fatalities for nondrivers using other modes of transportation that were less protective (mopeds, bicycles, and walking).	Cointervention: The study compared driving safety in 2 different countries with differences in traffic regulations and driving conditions. The reported numbers are not comprehensive because the data include only the number of accidents and fatalities that were reported by police.

Reference: Hakamies-Blomqvist, L., Johansson, K., & Lundburg, C. (1996). Medical screening of older drivers as a traffic safety measure: A comparative Finnish–Swedish evaluation study. *Journal of the American Geriatrics Society, 44,* 650–653.

Author/Year	Study Objectives	Level/Design/Participants	Intervention & Outcome Measures	Results	Limitations
Hing et al. (2003)	Evaluate the impact of passengers on the safety of older drivers	II—Cohort study Crash data from Kentucky State Police reports $N = 28,275$ for age group 65–74 years	No intervention; was an observational study Outcomes: ■ Crash data from the Kentucky State Police Reports for 1995–1998. Crashes involving drivers ages 65 and older (65–75 and 75+). ■ Single- and multi-vehicle crashes	Drivers older than age 75 were involved in crashes more often than drivers ages 65–74. Older women were involved in multi-vehicle crashes more often than men. Drivers with 2 or more passenger were more likely to be involved in crashes on roads with curves and grades, except during night driving.	Eye health and other factors were not included in the analysis. Authors did not examine the potential distractions that took place during driving, only the presence or absence of passengers.

Reference: Hing, J. Y. C., Stamatiadis, N., & Aultman-Hall, L. (2003). Evaluating the impact of passengers on the safety of older drivers. *Journal of Safety Research, 34,* 3343–3351.

| Ho et al. (2001) | Investigate the effects of age, clutter, and scene luminance on the identification of traffic signs | I—Randomized controlled trial

Experiment I: *N* = 28 (14 participants ages 56–71 and 14 participants ages 20–27)

Experiment II: *N* = 28 (14 participants ages 54–79 and 14 ages 18–30) | Experiment I: Images were classified on the basis of clutter (high/low and luminance (day/nighttime).

The participants were then asked to classify low-clutter daytime images and high-clutter daytime images, low-clutter nighttime images and high-clutter nighttime images

Experiment II: The images from Experiment I presented to participants, and the task was to identify whether traffic signs were present or absent in these images.

Outcomes:
- Error rate
- Reaction time
- Number of eye fixations
- Duration of last fixation
- Average fixation duration | The error rate was higher for the following:
- Older than younger drivers
- High-clutter than low-clutter trials
- Target-present trials than target-absent trials.

Reaction time was slower for the following:
- Older than younger drivers
- High-clutter trials than low-clutter trials
- Target-present than target-absent trials.

Eyes fixation was higher for the following:
- Older than younger drivers
- High-clutter than low-clutter trials
- Fixations for target-present trials than target-absent trials

Last fixation duration was longer for target-present trials than for target-absent trials.

Average fixation duration was longer for older than younger drivers. | Images were static and two dimensional, with no time limit, not mimicking the real-world driving situation and thus minimizing the applicability of the results. |

Reference: Ho, G., Scialfa, C. T., Caird, J. K., & Graw, T. (2001). Visual search for traffic signs: The effects of clutter, luminance, and aging. *Human Factors, 43,* 194–207.

(continued)

Author/Year	Study Objectives	Level/Design/Participants	Intervention & Outcome Measures	Results	Limitations
Imbeau et al. (1989)	Explore which of the instrument panel illumination colors, brightness, and character sizes are most suitable for night driving	II—Nonrandomized mixed-factorial design N = 24 (8 participants ages 19–30, 8 participants ages 31–50, and 8 participants ages 51–73)	All groups received interventions in a simulator laboratory ■ Chromaticity (blue green, green, orange, light blue, red, reddish orange, white, and amber) ■ Brightness (low and high) ■ Character size (1.5, 2.5, 3.7, and 5.5 mm) ■ Word complexity (low or high) Outcomes: ■ Response time: Stimulus presentation to a correct answer ■ Glance time: Length of time the participant looked before answering ■ Percentage of correct answers ■ Percentage of correct/incorrect answers ■ Lane deviation ■ Subjective opinion	There was a statistically significant difference between age groups. The smallest character size of 7 arcmin was reported to be difficult for older drivers to read and led to decrements in driving and word recognition. The 11 arcmin was good for younger and middle-age drivers, but older drivers still had degradation of driving. Although preference should be given to 25 arcmin, 17 arcmin is acceptable with adequate luminance. In addition, eye fixation and average fixation duration was higher in older than younger participants.	The result of the study might be masked because of interaction and/or confounding effect of several variables. Use of a simulator may limit generalizability of results to on-road driving.

Reference: Imbeau, D., Wierwille, W. W., Wolf, L. D., & Chun, G. A. (1989). Effects of instrument panel luminance and chromaticity on reading performance and preference in simulated driving. *Human Factors, 31,* 147–160.

Author/Year	Study Objectives	Level/Design/Participants	Intervention & Outcome Measures	Results	Limitations
Jacobs et al. (1997)	Determine the effectiveness of participation-oriented education in driving rehabilitation for older adults	I—Randomized controlled trial N = 21 participants older than age 55 who drive more than 1,000 miles/year	Group 1: Participants drove in a Doron Precision Systems driving simulator for 2 hr with films used in the simulator to provide education on proper driving techniques, crash avoidance techniques, and destination driving. Group 2: Participants watched the films taken from the driving simulator that provided education on proper driving techniques, crash avoidance techniques, and destination driving, for 1 hr. Group 3: No intervention	On-road performance for Group 1 was significantly higher compared with both Group 2 and Group 3 driving performance. No significant difference was reported in clinical evaluation of driving skills between any groups.	Small sample size could limit applicability of results; Hawthorne effect, as both Group 1 and Group 2 received more attention than Group 3; assessment of the driving skills might not be a sensitive method to determine changes among the three groups.

Jacobs et al.
(1997)
(continued)

Outcomes:
- On-road evaluation of driving skills that included starting/stopping, steering, position in lane, speed, turns, and braking reaction
- Clinical evaluation of driving skills such as motion/strength, grip, coordination, and proprioception
- Subjective improvement in driving confidence

Reference: Jacobs, K., Jennings, L., Forman, M., Benjamin, J., DiPanfilo, K., & LaPlante, M. (1997). The use of participation-oriented education in the rehabilitation of driving skills in older adults. *Work, 8,* 281–291.

| Janke (1994) | Determine whether California Mature Driver Improvement (MDI), a driving improvement course for older adults, had an effect on crash rates | II—Nonrandomized controlled trial

N = 564,444 MDI group: 197,452 participants with an average age of 69
Comparison group: 366,992 participants with an average age of 66 | MDI group received information on effects of visual and audio perception, fatigue, medications, and alcohol on driving performance and ways to compensate; updates on rules of the road and equipment; how to plan travel time and select routes for safety and efficiency; and how to make crucial decisions in dangerous, hazardous, and unforeseen situations. The total class duration was approximately 7 hr.

Comparison group received no intervention.

Outcomes:
■ Crash rates before taking the course, after 6 months, 18 months, and 30 months | Unadjusted comparison between the MDI and the control group indicated that there was no significant difference in terms of accident rates after 6, 18, and 30 months. Although the use of analysis of covariance for adjustment indicates that in 1 cohort there were fewer crashes in the MDI group and in the other cohort there were more, in the analysis using 2-state least-squares regression, completion of the MDI program was associated with more total and fatal injury crashes. Participants in the MDI group received fewer traffic citations in both analyses. | Lack of randomization to treatment.

The ability to show cause in the relationship is limited, because many variables were not controlled for in the analysis. |

Reference: Janke, M. K. (1994). *Mature Driver Improvement Program in California* (Transportation Research Record 1438). [Available from California Department of Motor Vehicles, Research and Development Section, 2415 First Avenue, Sacramento, CA 95818]

(continued)

Author/Year	Study Objectives	Level/Design/Participants	Intervention & Outcome Measures	Results	Limitations
Ker et al. (2003)	Determine the effectiveness of postlicense driver education in reducing motor vehicle accidents	I—Systematic review of the randomized controlled (Level I) trials about postlicense driver education N = 28 randomized trials reviewed	The method consisted of systematically selecting the Level I studies using the predefined criteria and analyzing them. Outcomes: ■ Traffic offenses ■ Motor vehicle crashes ■ Injuries (fatal and nonfatal)	The systematic review of randomized controlled trials provides no evidence that postlicense driver education programs are effective in preventing road traffic injuries or crashes. The results indicated a small reduction in the occurrence of traffic offenses with no differences in traffic and injury crashes.	Individual study limitations include inadequate allocation concealment, lack of blinding of outcome assessment, and large losses to follow-up. The results should be interpreted with caution because of heterogeneity in several meta-analyses due to differences in study populations and types of educational programs.

Reference: Ker, K., Roberts, I., Collier, T., Renton, F., & Bunn, F. (2003). Post-license driver education for the prevention of road traffic crashes. *Cochrane Database of Systematic Reviews, 3,*CD003734.

| Klavora et al. (1995) | Determine the efficacy of the Dynavision apparatus in improving psychomotor abilities and behind-the-wheel driving performance after stroke | III—Nonrandomized 1-group pretest–posttest

N = 10 participants ages 45–80 who had a stroke between 6 and 18 months before the study | Participants received Dynavision apparatus training for 6 weeks, 3 times per week, with each session lasting 20 min.

Dynavision was used to measure visual attention, visuomotor coordination, response time, peripheral awareness, eye scanning, concentration, simple cognitive processing, physical endurance, and combinations of these skills.

Outcome:
■ Behind-the-wheel (BTW) driving performance | Participants performed better on divided-attention and selected-attention tasks after training. Speed of processing did not improve with training.

On the BTW assessment, 60% of the participants earned a rating of "safe to resume driving" and/or to receive on-road driving lessons. This percentage of individuals gaining "safe" status after intervention was higher than the previously reported success rate of 24%. | Learning effect; Dynavision was used as a training as well as assessment tool.

The BTW assessment was reported to be very subjective, resulting in bias; lack of control group. |

Reference: Klavora, P., Gaskovski, P., Martin, K., Forsyth, R. D., Heslegrave, R. J., et al. (1995). The effects of dynavison rehabilitation on behind-the-wheel driving ability and selected psychomotor abilities of persons after stroke. *American Journal of Occupational Therapy, 49,* 534–542.

| Kline et al. (1999) | Whether the ability to identify optically blurred text could be affected by either daytime or nighttime conditions | I—Randomized controlled trial

Experiment I: N = 24 (12 participants ages 21–29 and 12 participants ages 55–71) Experiment II: N = 24 (12 participants ages 17–26 and 12 participants ages 58–78) | Experiment I: Participants looked at traffic signs under 3 levels of visual acuity and 2 luminance levels: daytime and nighttime

Experiment II: Participants looked at traffic and novel signs under 3 levels of visual acuity and 2 luminance levels: daytime and nighttime | Legibility thresholds were lower for older participants than younger participants. Also, familiar objects (standard signs) had lower thresholds than unfamiliar signs. Legibility was higher for daylight condition compared with nighttime. | Optical blurring of a sign that does not physically change size is not the same as physically increasing the distance between an observer and a sign. This makes it difficult to generalize the results to on-road driving. |

Kline et al. (1999) (continued)			Outcomes: ■ Acuity in diopters ■ Legibility	No significant difference in correction was required for both younger and older participants in both Experiments I and II.	

Reference: Kline, D. W., Buck, K., Sell, Y., Bolan, T. L., & Dewar, R. E. (1999). Older observers' tolerance of optical blur: Age differences in the identification of defocused text signs. *Human Factors, 41*, 356–364.

Koffman & Salstrom (2001)	Determine use of customer satisfaction surveys in improving fixed-route transportation services	III—Cross-sectional survey $N = 3$ separate transit agencies ($n1 = 14,963$; $n2 = 15,058$; $n3 = 1,399$)	No intervention; observational study Customer satisfaction survey: 2 agencies used on-board surveys, and 1 used telephone interviews to identify quality of services in terms of on-time performance, drivers, cleanliness, customer information, security, safety, and overall transit service. Also, 2 open-ended questions determined overall satisfaction with the services.	An impact analysis that identifies a satisfaction gap and identifies the impact of improving a given service was used; the results indicate that older adults feel that adding service would have the greatest impact on ridership, followed by drivers, reliable equipment, and on-time performance.	A limitation of cross-sectional surveys is that it is difficult to know the timing in the relationship of variables.

Reference: Koffman, D., & Salstrom, R. (2001). *How to best serve seniors on existing transit services* (No. MTI Report 01-04). San Jose, CA: San Jose State University, College of Business, Mineta Transportation Institute.

Kostyniuk et al. (1997)	Evaluate how older drivers used Tetra Star, an advanced-traveler information system	III—Pretest-posttest $N = 102$ (34 participants ages 19–29, 34 participants ages 30–64, and 34 participants ages 65–80)	Participants drove a project-lease vehicle for 28 days that was equipped with Tetra Star. Participants filled out daily logs and completed a usability survey that included questions on patterns of use, relative utility, and perceived ease of use.	Older drivers were less likely than other participants to use the Tetra Star system for commuting. In addition, older drivers took more of their trips in the morning than did younger drivers. Older drivers reported more difficulty with learning and using the destination-selection feature than younger drivers. Although older drivers had less difficulty understanding directions than younger drivers, older participants also reported that the information from the guidance system was presented too far in advance.	Lack of a control group.

Reference: Kostyniuk, L., Eby, D. W., Christoff, C., Hopp, M. L., & Streff, F. M. (1997). *The FAST-TRAC natural use leased-car study: An evaluation of user perceptions and behaviors of Ali-Scout by age and gender* (Report UMTRI-97-09). Ann Arbor: University of Michigan, Transportation Research Institute.

(continued)

Evidence Table *(continued)*

Author/Year	Study Objectives	Level/Design/Participants	Intervention & Outcome Measures	Results	Limitations
LaMotte et al. (2000)	Determine the effect of aftermarket tinting of rear and side windows on driving vision	II—Nonrandomized mixed-factor design *N* = 20 (10 participants ages 20–29 and 10 participants ages 60–69)	Tinted side windows either without aftermarket film 82% transmittance (control group), medium tints of 57% transmittance, or dark tints with 18% transmittance. Outcome: ■ Contrast sensitivity, which was measured for gratings at each of 6 spatial frequencies (0.5, 1, 2, 4, 8, and 12 cycles/degree)	For age group 20–29, contrast sensitivity between the control and dark tint was significant, as was contrast sensitivity between medium and dark tints. For age group 60–69, the medium tints reduce contrast sensitivity for middle and high spatial frequency.	Use of a nonstandardized instrument for measuring contrasts sensitivity and small sample size could minimize the applicability of the results to the overall population of elderly people.

Reference: LaMotte, J., Ridder III, W., Yeung, K., & De Land, P. (2000). Effect of aftermarket automobile window tinting films on driver vision. *Human Factors, 42,* 327–336.

| Laux (1991) | Determine effects of expectancy and age of drivers in terms of locations of vehicle controls and display systems | I—Randomized mixed-factorial design

N = 38 (16 participants ages 19–27 and 22 participants ages 60–87) | Drivers' expectancies for 14 controls and 4 displays were assessed first in the participant's car, and then participants were given 3 different cars to drive.

Outcomes:
■ Drivers' expectancy survey
■ Duration for locating controls/displays | Significant differences in terms of time for locating controls/displays were reported among the 3 vehicles and between age groups. Older participants were slower than younger ones to locate controls and displays. Older drivers were slower on controls/displays that they would likely not use or need in an everyday driving situation. | Study is of good quality. |

Reference: Laux, L. F. (1991). *Locating vehicle controls and displays: Effects of expectancy and age.* Washington, DC: AAA Foundation for Traffic Safety.

| Liu (2001) | Explore whether drivers' reactions and performance are affected by the multimodality display in ATIS and to explore differences in driving performance due to age of the driver. | I—Randomized mixed-factor design

N = 32 (16 participants ages 18–25 and 16 participants ages 65–73) | Both groups completed 6 driving scenarios (approximately 60 min) on a simulation with feedback: audio only, visual only, multimodality only, and driving (high- and low-load driving).

Outcomes:
■ Data from the simulator, including response time, number of missed button pushes, and total of correct turns.
■ Assessment by a rater on navigation-related errors, turn direction, and name of turn street.
■ Subjective Workload Assessment Technique and preference rating by drivers. | For both age groups, users of the multimodality display produced fewer misses than those in the auditory condition or the visual condition. The visual display accounted for the largest number of missed turns, and the multimodality display accounted for very few navigation-related errors. There was a significant difference in performance for older and younger groups for all study tasks. The results indicate that the visual display led to less safe driving, because it imposed higher demands on participants' attention. | Implementation of the results obtained from these experiments into a clinical protocol has not been clearly stated in the study, and its effectiveness might be questionable. |

Reference: Liu, Y-C. (2001). Comparative study of the effects of auditory, visual, and multimodality displays on drivers' performance in advanced traveller information systems. *Ergonomics, 44,* 425–442.

Llaneras et al. (1998)	Investigate the effectiveness of an ergonomic intervention in producing safe and productive driving in commercial vehicle drivers	I—Randomized controlled trial *N* = 107, ages 31–76 There were 5 age cohorts: (1) younger than 50, (2) 50–54, (3) 55–59, (4) 60–64, and (5) 65 and older.	Interventions evaluated included use of the Simulated Prescriptive Auditory Navigational System, which provided prescriptive routing information in the form of auditory commands versus traditional paper-based maps; training on visual search and scanning patterns; comparison of drivers with and without an on-board advanced auditory warning system; and comparison of drivers with an automatic transmission versus drivers with a manual transmission. There also was a control group with no intervention. Outcomes: ■ Number of missed turns, number of navigational queries, and time to complete the 10-mile (16-km) course ■ Visual search and mirror checks ■ Time of detection of malfunction ■ Manipulation of vehicle during curves, executing turns, speed adjustment, lane position, setting up for turns, overall driving, and braking	Drivers equipped with the Simulated Prescriptive Auditory Navigational System made fewer navigational errors and inquires than drivers who relied on paper-based maps and directions. In addition, drivers exposed to the visual search and scanning training program had better monitoring performance, as measured by visual search and mirror-check scores. Drivers provided with an auditory warning had significantly higher detection rates than drivers without the advanced warning system, and drivers whose trucks were equipped with automatic transmission had better performance during curves than their counterparts equipped with the manual transmission. Because the study was conducted in a laboratory setting, generalization to on-road vehicle driving environments is limited. Because all the participants in the experimental group were exposed to all 4 types of intervention, the effect of cointervention might exist, masking the true effect due to a particular intervention.

Reference: Llaneras, R. E., Swezey, R. W., Brock, J. F., Rogers, W. C., & Van Cott, H. P. (1998). Enhancing the safe driving performance of older commercial vehicle drivers. *International Journal of Industrial Ergonomics, 22,* 217–245.

(continued)

Evidence Table *(continued)*

Author/Year	Study Objectives	Level/Design/Participants	Intervention & Outcome Measures	Results	Limitations
Marshall et al. (2002)	Evaluate the rates of crashes and traffic violations among drivers with restricted licenses and compare the crash and traffic violation rates before and after driver restrictions were imposed	II—Cohort *N* = 703,758 (all Saskatchewan drivers registered from January 1992 to April 1999)	No intervention; this was an observational study in which all the drivers with either driving and/or licensure restriction were followed for 4 years after imposition. Outcome: ■ Number of crashes and traffic violations resulting in insurance claim collected from database of Saskatchewan government insurance	Drivers with restricted driving and licensure were reported to have significantly lower rate of accidents and traffic violations but a higher risk of at-fault crashes compared with drivers with unrestricted driving access. After restrictions were imposed, there was a significant reduction, by 12.8%, in the number of crashes per 1,000 drivers/week. Finally, when the comparison was made in number of crashes after 4 years of imposition to that before imposition, a significant reduction was observed.	Only crashes with insurance claims were included in the study, which might not be a comprehensive inclusion representing all incidences. Because the study was observational in nature, there was no control of the study over improving compliance of drivers with restrictions. The study did not control for the medical diagnosis or disability, which might have affected some of the outcomes.

Reference: Marshall, S. C., Spasoff, R., Nair, R., & Walraven, C. (2002). Restricted driver licensing for medical impairments: Does it work? *Canadian Medical Association Journal, 167,* 747–751.

Author/Year	Study Objectives	Level/Design/Participants	Intervention & Outcome Measures	Results	Limitations
Mazer et al. (2001)	Examine the use of the UFOV visual attention analyzer in the evaluation and retraining of visual attention skills in clients with stroke	III—Pretest–posttest design *N* = 6 Mean age: 60; range: 36–82 Participants comprised a large group of 52, from which the 6 were the first to volunteer to participate in training program	Training using the UFOV visual attention analyzer for 20 sessions focusing on 3 modules: (1) processing speed, (2) divided attention, and (3) selective attention. Outcome: ■ UFOV visual attention analyzer: Visual attention composed of processing speed, divided attention, and selective attention	Significant improvement from pretest in 2 domains of visual attention—divided attention and selective attention—was reported for all participants. In terms of processing speed, even though there was improvement after posttest compared with pretest, it was not significantly different.	Cointervention: Participants were receiving other forms of intervention. Temporal positive/negative effects of stroke were not taken into consideration. Learning effects from using the UFOV visual field analyzer for both training and for assessment; small sample size; lack of control group.

Reference: Mazer, B. L., Sofer, S., Korner-Bitensky, N., & Gelinas, I. (2001). Use of the UFOV to evaluate and retrain visual attention skills in clients with stroke: A pilot study. *American Journal of Occupational Therapy, 55,* 552–557.

Mazer et al. (2003)	Compare the effectiveness of the UFOV visual attention retraining and conventional visuoperception treatment on the driving performance of clients with stroke	I—Randomized controlled block design *N* = 97; mean age: 66	Intervention: Training for 20 sessions using the UFOV visual attention analyzer. Control: Conventional computerized visuoperception retraining for 20 sessions Outcomes: ■ UFOV: Measures speed of visual processing, divided attention, and selected attention. ■ On-road driving evaluation, including driving behaviors, knowledge, and application of driving regulations. ■ Visuoperception: Included the Complex Reaction Timer; Motor-Free Visual Perception Test; Single and Double Letter Cancellation Test; Money Road Map Test of Direction Sense; Trail Making Test, Parts A and B; Bells Test; and Charron Test	No significant difference in visuoperceptual functioning was reported between the experimental and control groups. Although an improvement in driving performance was noted for the intervention group, the difference did not approach statistical significance. There was, however, an almost twofold increase (52.4% vs. 28.6%) in the rate of success on the on-road driving evaluation after UFOV training for participants with right-sided lesions	Cointervention: Participants were receiving other forms of intervention Learning effects from using the UFOV visual field analyzer for both training and for assessment.

Reference: Mazer, B. L., Sofer, B., Korner-Bitensky, N., Gelinas, I., Hanley, J., & Wood-Dauphinee, S. (2003). Effectiveness of a visual attention retraining program on the driving performance of clients with stroke. *Archives of Physical Medicine and Rehabilitation, 84.*

McKnight & McKnight (1992)	Evaluate the effectiveness of in-vehicle navigation systems in enhancing safety by reducing the distraction involved in looking at maps and searching for street signs	Level I—Randomized mixed-factor design *N* = 150 (50 participants under age 25, 50 participants ages 25–50, and 50 participants over age 50)	Video-based simulation evaluated driver performance using 5 alternative navigation information sources: (1) area map, (2) strip map, (3) strip map with position indicator, (4) directional guidance with an audible signal, and (5) a combination of position indication and directional guidance. Outcomes: ■ Total time looking at navigation displays ■ Appropriate traffic responses	The results indicate that older drivers failed to anticipate turns more frequently and had a higher cumulative glance duration than younger participants. The guidance system, which produced an alarm and a directional arrow before a turn, had the lowest error rate and total looking time but was ranked as least preferred of the navigational displays.	Use of a simulator limits the ability to generalize to on-road driving.

Reference: McKnight, J. A., & McKnight, A. S. (1992). *The effects of in-vehicle navigation information systems upon driver attention.* Washington, DC: American Automotive Association Foundation for Traffic Safety.

(continued)

Author/Year	Study Objectives	Level/Design/Participants	Intervention & Outcome Measures	Results	Limitations
Mollenhauer, Dingus, & Hulse (1995)	Investigate the efficacy of in-vehicle technologies integrated into a heads-up display (HUD) to help elderly drivers compensate for age-related degradation in driving performance.	II—Nonrandomized mixed-factor design $N = 32$ (16 participants ages 65–69 and 16 participants ages 70 and older)	To navigate from one destination to another (while doing tasks such as finding street cross sections, following vehicles, and passing vehicles) using either a paper map or a HUD under 2 types of conditions: (1) baseline events and (2) navigation with braking Outcomes: ■ Driving performance ■ Navigation performance measures: Number of correct turns and navigation time ■ Collision avoidance performance measures ■ Subjective Workload Assessment Technique: Measuring mental workload	Drivers had more correct turns when using HUD compared with the standard display and paper map. Subjective Workload Assessment Technique: No significant difference in mental workload was reported between HUD display and standardized display. Results from a satisfaction questionnaire indicated that the older adults would use an integrated HUD.	Impact of the HUD on other aspects, such as attention and confusion, was not reported; generalization of the outcomes to real-world driving situation may be limited.

Reference: Mollenhauer, M. A., Dingus, T. A., & Hulse, M. C. (1995). *The potential for advanced vehicle systems to increase the mobility of elderly drivers.* Iowa City: University of Iowa, Public Policy Center.

Author/Year	Study Objectives	Level/Design/Participants	Intervention & Outcome Measures	Results	Limitations
Ostrow et al. (1992)	Determine the effectiveness of a joint range of motion exercise program on improving driving abilities in older adults.	I—Randomized control trial $N = 38$ drivers ages 60–85; 22 in the intervention group and 16 in the control group	Intervention group: Upper-body (including neck) range of motion, stretching exercise for 8 weeks at home Control group: Instruction in the car for improving driving skills Outcomes: ■ Range-of-motion tests ■ Automobile Driver On-Road Performance Test ■ Behavioral recording log	Improvement in trunk rotation and shoulder flexibility was reported in the intervention group compared with the control group. Participants in the experimental group improved on handling position and observing compared with the control group. No difference, however, was reported between the groups in terms of amount of driving per week.	Attention bias: Intervention group received more attention than control group.

Reference: Ostrow, A. C., Shafran, P., & McPherson, K. (1992). The effects of a joint range-of-motion physical fitness training program on the automobile driving skills of older adults. *Journal of Safety Research, 23,* 207–219.

Author/Year	Study Objectives	Level/Design/Participants	Intervention & Outcome Measures	Results	Limitations
Owsley et al. (2002)	Determine the efficacy and effectiveness of cataract surgery on crashes and driving performance of older adults	II—Prospective cohort study $N = 277$ patients with cataracts, ages 55–84	Intervention condition: Participants received cataract surgery and intraocular lens implantation	The intervention group was reported to have half the crash rate (0.47) compared with the control group, after adjusting for race, visual	The study considered only police-reported incidents, which may be a limited representation of the total accident crashes that occurred.

Owsley et al. (2002) (continued)			Control condition: No cataract surgery Outcome: ■ Number of motor vehicle crashes as reported by police	acuity, and contrast sensitivity. The study also reported a reduced number of crashes after cataract surgery, with a number of 4.74 per million miles of travel.	

Reference: Owsley, C., McGwin, G., Jr., Sloane, M., Wells, J., Stalvey, V. T., & Gauthreaux, S. (2002). Impact of cataract surgery on motor vehicle crash involvement by older adults. *Journal of the American Medical Association, 7,* 841–849.

Pohlmann & Treankle (1994)	Investigate the effectiveness of the TRAVELPILOT navigational system in improving navigation performance, driving performance, and reducing mental workload in older drivers	II—Nonrandomized mixed-factor design *N* = 48 (24 participants ages 35–50 and 24 participants ages 61–70)	All the participants received 3 forms of intervention: (1) use of TRAVELPILOT navigational system, (2) use of map, and (3) experimenter giving directions Outcomes: ■ Driving performance ■ Navigation system operation ■ Effectiveness of (personal) navigation ■ Computer Anxiety Rating Scale	Participants in both age groups were significantly more likely to have slight and severe lane deviations when using TRAVELPILOT than in the road map condition (*p* < .001). The lane deviations that occurred while using TRAVELPILOT were reported to result in a high accident risk due to the requirement of turning the head to fixate on the display or compensatory reactions when turning the head to one side and steering to another. No difference in regard to mental workload imposed by the different systems was reported. Also, the acceptance rate for the navigation system was similar for both age groups.	Lack of randomization

Reference: Pohlmann, S., & Traenkle, U. (1994). Orientation in road traffic. Age-related differences using an in-vehicle navigation system and a conventional map. *Accident Analysis and Prevention, 26,* 689–702.

(continued)

Evidence Table (continued)

Author/Year	Study Objectives	Level/Design/Participants	Intervention & Outcome Measures	Results	Limitations
Riedel et al. (1998)	Investigate effects of Piracetam on driving performance of elderly individuals without dementia	I—Randomized crossover trial $N = 38$ drivers between ages 60 and 80; mean age: 66.9	Oral administration of the drug Piracetam twice daily for 4 weeks. Compliance with the protocol was determined by testing urine at Days 2 and 28. Control component: Placebo Outcomes: ■ Driving performance: Lateral deviation ■ Balance: Sway and postural stability	Significant improvement in the intervention treatment period was observed with lower lateral deviation compared with placebo period. Improvement in sway was observed in participants after 4 weeks on Piracetam compared with the control period. No adverse effects were observed with the use of the drug.	Driving performance was not comprehensive; period of treatment with Piracetam may not have been long enough to determine the full effect of the drug.

Reference: Riedel, W. J., Peters, M. L. Van Boxtel, M. P. J., & O'Hanlon, J. F. (1998). The influence of Piracetam on actual driving behaviour of elderly subjects. *Human Psychopharmacology, 13,* 108–114.

Author/Year	Study Objectives	Level/Design/Participants	Intervention & Outcome Measures	Results	Limitations
Roenker et al. (2003)	Determine effectiveness of the speed-of-processing training in UFOV on driving performance	I—Randomized controlled trial $N = 104$ licensed drivers Mean age: 69; range: 48–94	Group 1: Control group with no intervention ($n = 27$) Group 2: Speed-of-processing training with individual UFOV on a computer screen ($n = 51$) Group 3: Simulator training, focusing on crash avoidance, managing intersections, and scanning ($n = 26$) Outcome: ■ Open-road driving evaluation. All assessments were completed pre- and postintervention and 18 months after intervention	Although the data indicate that improvement in driving skill is specific to type of training, improvement was observed in all 3 groups, with Group 3 improving the most compared with the control and speed-of-processing training groups. Some gains disappeared at 18 months, but retention of the driving skills acquired during training was maintained in the speed-of-processing training group after 18 months.	Lack of assessment of cognitive function.

Reference: Roenker, D. L., Cissell, G. L., Ball, K. K., Wadley, V. G., & Edwards, J. D. (2003). Speed-of-processing and driving simulator training result in improved driving performance. *Human Factors, 45,* 218–233.

Author/Year	Study Objectives	Level/Design/Participants	Intervention & Outcome Measures	Results	Limitations
Sayer et al. (1999)	Investigate the potential benefits of hydrophobic treatment on the driver-side window and exterior rearview mirror on improving distance judgment for drivers	I—Randomized mixed factor $N = 24$ (12 participants ages 20–28 and 12 participants ages 66–83)	4 experimental conditions with treated/untreated mirrors and windows. Water was used to simulate a rain effect. Outcome: ■ Distance estimation	There was no difference in distance estimates to target vehicle with the application of hydrophobic treatment to the driver-side window and exterior rearview mirror for older and younger participants.	The study determined only perception of the distance from target vehicle, which may not be an actual measure of driving performance.

Reference: Sayer, J. R., Mefford, M. L., Flannagan, M. J., & Sivak, M. (1999). *The effects of hydrophobic treatment of the driver-side window and rearview mirror on distance judgment* (Report No. UMTRI-99-22). Ann Arbor: University of Michigan, Transportation Research Institute.

Schmidt et al. (1991)	Investigate the effects of Piracetam on the driving performance of drivers with reduced reaction capacity	I—Randomized controlled trial *N* = 96 participants ages 48–76 49 intervention; 47 control	Intervention group: Participants were given 4.8g/day of Piracetem for 6 weeks Control group: Placebo Outcomes: ■ Driving test ■ Emotionality inventory (EMI–B)	A significant improvement after 6 weeks of intervention was reported in the intervention group in all areas of driving performance.	Long-term benefits/adverse effects of the drug are not reported in the study, which might be needed to determine the risk–benefit ratio.

Reference: Schmidt, U., Brendemuhl, D., Engels, K., Schenk, N., & Ludemann, E. (1991). Piracetam in elderly motorists. *Pharmacopsychiatry, 24*, 121–126.

Schumann et al. (1997)	Determine the effects of windshield rake angle and dashboard reflectance on different veiling glare and driving performance and object detection	I—Randomized controlled trial *N* = 16 (8 participants ages 18–30 and 8 participants ages 66–76)	9 combinations of 3 rake angles and 3 dashboard reflectances were presented with 2 levels of contrast of pedestrian. Outcomes: ■ Detection time: Time required to detect pedestrian ■ Missed response: Detection time of more than 5 s was considered a missed response	Both windshield rake (mounting) angle and dashboard reflectance had measurable effects on visual performance, and effects were particularly pronounced if there was a large rake angle combined with high dashboard reflectance. Although there was no significant difference in detection time between the 2 age groups, the missed-response rate was higher for elderly participants compared with younger participants.	Other extraneous variables, such as dashboard gloss, texture, and inclination angle, which might have some influence on veiling glare, were not controlled for.

Reference: Schumann, J., Flannagan, M. J., Sivak, M., & Traube, E. C. (1997). Daytime veiling glare and driver visual performance: Influence of windshield rake angle and dashboard reflectance. *Journal of Safety Research, 28*, 133–146.

Shipp (1998)	Determine the impact of vision-related relicensing policies on traffic fatalities in the United States	II—Cohort study *N* = 49 state licensing entities	Observational study; no intervention was provided. Outcome: ■ State-level occupant fatalities as reported by the Fatal Accident Reporting System	Although there was no statistically significant difference for the relationship between vision testing policies in relicensing and number of fatalities, when adjusting for nonvision policies and nonpolicy factors (age, gender, socioeconomic status, population density, and environment), there was a significant difference in number of fatalities.	The Fatal Accident Reporting System database provides only number of deaths and not number of incidents.

Reference: Shipp, M. D. (1998). Potential human and economic cost-savings attributable to vision testing policies for driver license renewal, 1989–1991. *Optometry and Vision Science, 75*, 103–118.

(continued)

Evidence Table (continued)

Author/Year	Study Objectives	Level/Design/Participants	Intervention & Outcome Measures	Results	Limitations
Stalvey & Owsley (2003)	Evaluate the efficacy of Knowledge Enhances Your Safety in preventing crashes while driving in older individuals with visual limitations.	I—Randomized controlled trial *N* = 365 high-risk drivers older than age 60 with a visual acuity and/or processing deficit, high level of driving exposure, and a history of crash involvement Mean age: 74; range: 60–91	Group 1: Eye examination with discussion about impact of visual limitations of driving (*n* = 171) Group 2: Usual care plus educational intervention (2 sessions for 3 hr total; *n* = 194) Outcome: ■ The Driver Perceptions and Practices Questionnaire, which assessed self-perception of vision impairment and its impact on driving; perceived threat of crash involvement; barriers to the performance; benefits to the performance of self-regulatory practices; level of readiness to adopt new behavior; and regulatory self-efficacy	Perception for level of vision impairment and understanding about its impact on driving was higher in intervention group compared with control group. Perceived benefits of self-regulation and readiness to change was significantly higher in the intervention group compared with the control group. No significant difference was reported between groups in terms of perceived threat of crash involvement, perceived barriers to self-regulation, and perceived regulatory self-efficacy.	Outcomes are self-reported.

Reference: Stalvey, B. T., & Owsley, C. (2003). The development and efficacy of a theory-based educational curriculum to promote self-regulation among high-risk older drivers. *Health Promotion Practice, 4,* 109–119.

Author/Year	Study Objectives	Level/Design/Participants	Intervention & Outcome Measures	Results	Limitations
Staplin et al. (2003)	Evaluate the effectiveness of functional capacity evaluations to predict at-fault crashes in older adults	II—Cohort study *N* = 1,876 drivers from Maryland, ages 55 and older, who were randomly selected and then volunteered to participate	Participants were administered the Motor-Free Visual Perception Test Visual Closure subtest; Trail Making Test, Part B; delayed recall evaluation; useful field of view, Subtest 2; rapid pace walk; and head–neck rotation evaluation. Outcome: ■ Number of at-fault crashes at 2-year follow-up (1 year of additional data from earlier follow-up)	Motor-Free Visual Perceptual Test—Visual Closure subtest, Delayed Recall and Head–Neck Rotation were more valuable in predicting crashes shortly after the tests were administered and decreased predicability as time wore on. Trail-Making Test Part B and Rapid Pace Walk were still predictive of crashes 1 year beyond test administration. The results indicate that it is difficult to predict long-term driving performance based on specific cognitive–perceptual measures.	Limiting the outcome measure to at-fault crashes may be an inadequate predictor of the effect of cognitive and perceptual status.

Reference: Staplin, L., Gish, K. W., & Wagner, E. K. (2003). MaryPODS revisited: Updated crash analysis and implications for screening program implementation. *Journal of Safety Research, 34,* 389–397.

Author (Year)	Objective	Design/Sample	Methods/Outcomes	Results	Limitations
Steinfeld & Green (1995)	Examine driver performance with a simulated heads-up display (HUD) that might be used for navigation as compared to a conventional instrument panel (IP) display.	Level I—Randomized mixed-factors design. $N = 12$. 6 younger (18–30, mean age, 21) (M-3, F-3). 6 older (65+ years, mean age, 73) (M-3, F-3).	In 15 blocks of trials (practice and test), participants sitting in an automobile mock-up were presented with a slide of a road scene concurrently with a slide of a navigation system display appearing either on IP or HUD. The driver compared the two images and pressed either "same" or "different" on key on right-hand armrest. Outcomes: ▪ Response times (to nearest millisecond) ▪ Errors	While the response times of older drivers overall were longer compared to younger drivers, both groups had significantly shorter response times using HUD than IP.	Small sample size. Use of simulator may make it difficult to relate results to on-road conditions.

Reference: Steinfeld, A. & Green, P. (1995). *Driver response times to full-windshield heads-up displays for navigation and vision enhancement* (Technical Report UMTRI-95-29). Ann Arbor: University of Michigan, Transportation Research Institute.

Author (Year)	Objective	Design/Sample	Methods/Outcomes	Results	Limitations
Tan & Lerner (1995)	Evaluate a variety of auditory warnings that could be used in crash avoidance systems	Level I—Randomized mixed-factor design. $N = 32$ (16 participants ages 20–40 and 16 participants ages 65 and older)	28 auditory warnings were presented in a simulator while participants heard 2 levels of vehicle noise (truck and sedan). Auditory warnings were presented at 6 dB (A) above the vehicle noise level. Participants judged each sound for preference on a Likert scale.	4 warnings were preferred and include a low-fuel warning (a rapid siren) and a continuous, low-pitch ambulance siren. Overall, older listeners preferred all sounds more than younger participants. Older adults rated 4 sounds lower, and the authors report that age-induced hearing loss may have affected the perception of these sounds.	Generalization of the outcomes to real-world driving situation may be limited.

Reference: Tan, A. K., & Lerner, N. D. (1995). *Multiple attribute evaluation of auditory warning signals for in-vehicle crash avoidance systems* (Report DOT HS-808-535). Washington, DC: U.S. Department of Transportation, National Highway Traffic Safety Administration.

Author (Year)	Objective	Design/Sample	Methods/Outcomes	Results	Limitations
Vollrath et al. (2002)	Determine whether the presence of passengers when driving in a vehicle increases the risk of a collision with another vehicle	II—Nonrandomized population-based cohort design. $N = 112,847$ crashes to drivers older than age 18. Excluded single-vehicle crashes and those in which one involved was not a private car.	No intervention; observational study. Outcomes: ▪ Accidents reported by police ▪ Demographics of drivers ▪ Accident situational conditions (e.g., time of accident, weather conditions.) ▪ Description of accidents (e.g., cause, nature.)	The presence of passengers was a "protection" against accident risks for all age groups. This protection was reported to be most effective for drivers in the 50+ age group, followed by drivers ages 25–49, and was minimally effective for drivers ages 18–24. From the situational variables, visual conditions and traffic density influenced the passenger effect, whereas type of road and day of week did not show a significant influence.	The study did not consider the physical/mental condition of drivers, which needs to be controlled to examine complete effect of presence of passenger on accident risks.

Reference: Vollrath, M., Meilinger, T., & Kruger, H. (2002). How the presence of passengers influences the risk of a collision with another vehicle. *Accident Analysis and Prevention, 34,* 654–694.

(continued)

Evidence Table (continued)

Author/Year	Study Objectives	Level/Design/Participants	Intervention & Outcome Measures	Results	Limitations
Wolffsohn et al. (1997)	Determine the influence of cognition and age on factors such as accommodation, detection rate, and response times when using a car head-up display (HUD).	II—Nonrandomized mixed-factor design $N = 24$ drivers (8 participants ages 19–24, 8 participants ages 35–44, and 8 participants ages 49–74)	All 3 age groups received 3 types of cognitively demanding tasks: (1) low, (2) medium, and (3) high. Outcomes: ■ Accommodative response ■ Response time to changes in outside world and HUD images ■ Detection rate of changes in outside and HUD images ■ Subjective opinion about perceived task difficulty	With increase in cognitive demands there was increase in accommodative response in all age groups. The accommodative response was significantly different for day and night situations. A significant increase in response time was reported with an increase in cognitive demands for all age groups.	Lack of randomization.

Reference: Wolffsohn, J. S., McBrien, N. A., Edgar, K., & Stout, T. (1997). The influence of cognition and age on accommodation, detection rate, and response times when using a car head-up display (HUD). *Ophthalmic and Physiological Optics, 18,* 243–253.

Author/Year	Study Objectives	Level/Design/Participants	Intervention & Outcome Measures	Results	Limitations
Yee & Melichar (1992)	Develop and evaluate the effectiveness of a 3-level multiphasic integrated assessment and intervention strategy	II—Nonrandomized controlled trial $N = 254$ (174 intervention, 80 control) Mean age: 64; age range: 43–89	Intervention group ($n = 174$) completed the Older Driver Self-Assessment Inventory, which included 3 steps: 1. Identification of drivers potentially at risk through screening 2. Educational intervention improving knowledge and skills about driving 3. Driving simulation to remediate driving skills deficits Control group ($n = 80$) Outcome: ■ Attitudes Assessment Test (AAT) 18 questions that examine attitudes regarding driving and driver reeducation ■ Knowledge Assessment Test—31 questions included those regarding information on general driving, rules of the road, response to driving, and aging and driving conditions.	No differences in subjective opinion about perceived task difficulty were reported. There was no difference in attitudes between the pre- and posttest scores of the treatment and control groups. A pre–post test change for knowledge items on the KAT was noted only for participants who had the assessment and education components. There was a difference, however, in scores, depending on the location of instruction (Texas and California).	The use of multiple sites, types of participants, and multiple levels of intervention (with differential dropout rates of each) adds to the intervention bias. Because of the lack of a follow-up period, the long-term benefits of the Older Driver Self-Assessment Inventory in identification and remediation of older drivers in prevention of crashes are unknown.

Reference: Yee, D., & Melichar, J. F. (1992). *Accident prevention through driving skills assessment and interventions for older drivers: ApProgramme* (EDRS 371-127; CE 066-474). San Francisco: San Francisco State University.

Appendix D.
Infrastructure Design Summary

Adapted by Paula Bohr, PhD, OTR/L, FAOTA, from Staplin, L., Lococo, K., Byington, S., & Harkey, D. (2001). *Highway design handbook for older drivers and pedestrians* (Pub. No. FHWA-RD-01-103). Washington, DC: U.S. Department of Transportation, Federal Highway Administration.

Intersections

Skew

Intersecting roadways should meet at a 90° angle to allow for

- Optimal conditions to detect and make judgments about on-coming vehicles
- Increased maneuvering time for navigation of the intersection. This is especially important because of the decline in head and neck mobility and decrease in peripheral field that accompanies aging.

Design for Turns

- Wider turning lanes can facilitate better positioning of the vehicle within the lane in preparation for turning.
- Wider receiving lanes minimize the chances of encroachment on other lanes (i.e., swinging too wide to lengthen the turning radius and minimize rotation of the steering wheel).
- Wider lanes allow older drivers more opportunity to remain within the boundaries of their assigned lanes during turning maneuvers secondary to the diminished ability to share attention and to turn the steering wheel sharply enough, given their traveling speed, to negotiate the turn.
- For left turns, raised channelization, treated with retroreflective markings to increase visibility, provides additional cuing to older drivers who experience the age-related decline in visual acuity and

contrast sensitivity that impairs their abilities to detect or recognize pavement lane markings.

- Retroreflective pavement markings, used to indicate the turning path, provide additional cuing to minimize encroachment on other lanes.
- Wider lanes, raised channelization, and retroreflective pavement markings are especially important for high-traffic areas or ones where there is a demonstrated crash problem.
- Right-turn movements are facilitated by an adequate curb radius that minimizes the chance of hitting the curb. The size of the curb radius affects the size of vehicle that can turn at the intersections. As older drivers may drive larger cars, the curve radius needs to be adequate not only to avoid hitting the curb but also so that the driver does not encroach on other lanes of traffic while maneuvering around the corner.
- Lane use devices should provide enough preview time so that the older driver is less prone to erratic maneuvers such as lane weaving that result from late detection.
- Lane use control signs for lane assignment on intersection approach should be consistently positioned overhead on signal mast arms or span wire where they are more easily viewed. Pavement markings indicating lane use should be positioned in advance of the signalized intersection.

Design for Roundabouts

- Modern roundabouts are useful to address the problems that older drivers may have judging speeds and gaps to maneuver through turns.
- Roundabouts eliminate left turns, facilitate traffic flow, provide a large curb radius to improve maneuverability and reduce speed of vehicles entering the circle, thereby simplifying the decision-making process for the older driver.

Sight Distance Requirements

- An unobstructed view of the entire intersection and sufficient lengths of roadway give the older driver more time to make decisions about whether to proceed, slow, or stop to avoid a collision with potentially conflicting vehicles.
- Turning maneuvers require longer sight distance requirements for the older driver, as it may take significantly longer to perceive that a vehicle is moving closer at a constant speed before making a decision about whether to proceed with the turn.
- Sight distance can be increased for left turns by a positive offset of opposing left-turn lanes. This provides a margin of safety for older drivers who do not position themselves within the intersection before initiating a left turn.

Signage and Markings

Lane Delineations

- Signs indicating DIVIDED HIGHWAY CROSSING, WRONG WAY, DO NOT ENTER, KEEP RIGHT, AND ONE WAY should be oversized and treated with retroreflective sheeting to increase their conspicuity and legibility by older drivers. The use of retroreflective pavement markings indicating the turn path and retroreflective wrong-way arrows in the through lanes reduce the likelihood of entering the wrong lane.
- Retroreflective treatment applied to median noses increases their visibility and provides the older driver with more cues to assist their understanding of the intersection design.

Edgelines, Curbs, Medians, and Obstacles

- Marking curbs, medians and obstacles on their vertical face and a portion of the top surface decreases the likelihood of collision with the raised surfaces by making them more conspicuous to older drivers who may have decreased contrast sensitivity, reduced useful field of vision, increased decision time, and slower vehicle control movement execution.

Street Name Signs

- Street name identification signs must be detected and legible if they are to provide guidance to drivers.
- Detection is improved by placement of the sign and contrast of the sign with the surrounding background. For example, at major intersections, street name signs should be overhead mounted, as overhead signs are more likely to be seen before those located on either side of the roadway.
- Redundant signage in the form of advance street name signs, with black lettering on a yellow sign panel, should be placed upstream of the intersection at the midblock location.
- Detection is less of a problem on streets with lower volumes of traffic and where traffic speeds do not exceed 25 mph. In these cases, post-mounted street name signs may be used, but a minimum letter height of 6" should be used to accommodate the reduced visual acuity associated with increasing age.
- Legibility of signs is improved with larger lettering of signs, more luminance (brightness) of the characters, and positive contrast between the letters and the sign.
- Retroreflective treatments that increase sign conspicuity and legibility at the widest available observation angles accommodate the older drivers who experience age-related visual acuity loss.
- Using mixed-case fonts with more character openness and smaller inter-character spacing such as the Clearview font improves legibility distance. Additionally, using larger letter height fonts (30% larger than standard highway character size) allow older drivers to read the signs far enough in advance of the intersection to make decisions about negotiating the intersection. If necessary, borders around standard panel size signs can be eliminated to increase legibility.

ONE-WAY and WRONG-WAY Signs

- Older drivers who have difficulty abstracting information and making quick decisions often require more effective and more conspicuous signs to alert them to wrong-way movements.

- Accommodation for the age differences in glare sensitivity and restricted peripheral vision should be provided through provision of multiple or advance signs as well as changes in size, luminance, and placement of signs.
- Wider intersections, especially divided roadways, require additional ONE WAY signs be placed on the divider median to increase conspicuity. Additionally, DO NOT ENTER and WRONG WAY signs may be needed. Retroreflective treatments increase visibility of signs, and high contrast provides better legibility.

STOP and YIELD Intersection Signs

- Age-related deficits in vision and attention necessitate improved stop control and yield control at non-signalized intersections.
- At intersections where greater visibility or emphasis is needed, the STOP sign size (standard 30") should be increased to 36", while the YIELD sign size (standard 36") should be increased to 48".
- Background retroreflective levels for STOP and YIELD signs should be sufficient to provide conspicuity and timely detection.
- Rumble strips or transverse pavement stripping upstream of the stop-controlled intersection serve as an alert when sight restrictions or high approach speeds are present. Additionally, a STOP AHEAD sign can be installed to provide a minimum preview distance and ensure adequate time to stop.

Traffic Control Signals

Traffic Signals

- Older drivers need increased signal luminance (brightness) and contrast to perceive traffic signals. Performance of the older driver also may suffer because of disabling glare.
- A wide viewing angle of the signal helps to increase the signal strength, as information is accessible over longer intervals.

- A large, black surround behind the signal (backplate) provides improved contrast, especially where there is potential for sun glare problems.
- Intervals between phases should be based on perception–reaction time, with a longer yellow interval to accommodate older drivers.

For left-turn movements:

- Protected-only operations, ideally leading protected left turns, are recommended to reduce the crash rates of elderly people at signalized intersections.
- Overhead LEFT TURN YIELD ON GREEN signs alert drivers to the signal, and redundant signs indicating left turn AT SIGNAL, positioned at an adequate preview distance before the intersection, allows the driver to position the vehicle in the left-turn lane.
- Because older drivers often have difficulty integrating time and distance information to estimate approaching vehicle speeds, it is important that the timing of the left turn signal be of sufficient length to provide adequate decision-making (go/no go) time for the older driver.
- The green-arrow signal light should terminate into a yellow before going to a steady red to allow a buffer for slower moving vehicles to complete the turn across on-coming traffic lanes before that traffic begins to enter the intersection.

For right-turn movements:

- Right-turn-on-red should be prohibited at intersections where the skew of the intersecting roadways limits sight distance. This is particularly important for older drivers whose restricted head and neck motion place them at a disadvantage for perceiving approaching conflicting traffic.
- When right turns are not permitted, a steady circular red indicator should be used along with a NO TURN ON RED sign positioned overhead, where it is most conspicuous.
- When right turns are permitted, the stop line for the right-turn lane should be offset 6–10 feet forward of the other lanes to provide better sight

distance. Additionally, TURNING TRAFFIC MUST YIELD TO PEDESTRIANS signs should be used at intersections where turning vehicles conflict with pedestrians who are using the crosswalk.

Fixed Lighting

- Fixed lighting on a roadway increases the visibility of the roadway and the immediate surrounding area. Roadway lighting permits drivers to maneuver more safely and efficiently, particularly where there are shifting lane alignments, turn-only lane assignments, pavement width transitions that force a path following adjustment, or at intersections.
- Maintenance of lighting installations should include cleaning lamp lenses regularly and replacing the lenses when their output falls below 80% of peak performance.

Interchanges

Exits From Highways

Exit Signing

- Exit signs must be detectable and legible to be effective. Redundant overhead placement of exit signs upstream from the exit ramp facilitates detection. Retroreflective treatments increase sign conspicuity and legibility to accommodate the drivers with age-related visual acuity loss.
- As with overhead street signs, the use of mixed case fonts with more character openness and smaller inter-character spacing (e.g., Clearview) improves legibility distance. Mixed-case fonts such as Clearview also should be used for ground-mounted signs to increase reading distance of all highway destination signs.
- The use of larger letters aids the older driver in reading unfamiliar words or word combinations. To minimize confusion, arrow shafts appearing on upstream diagrammatic guide signs should match the number of lanes on the roadway at the sign's location.

Ramp Gore Delineation

- *Gore* is defined as the area immediately beyond where two roadways split, bounded by the edges of those roadways.
- When the exit is not illuminated or partially illuminated, the gore should be marked with partially retroreflective flexible posts and partially retroreflective pavement markers to assist drivers in identifying the boundaries of the exit lane. Especially at night, when drivers cannot rely on a direct view of the ramp, these markers provide an outline of the location of the gore.
- For older drivers with limited night vision, the partially retroreflective flexible posts are more effective than other types of markers.

Acceleration/Deceleration Lane Design

- Diminished capabilities to accurately and reliably integrate speed and perceived distance information for moving vehicles, reduced neck or trunk flexibility, and age-related deficits in attention sharing capabilities place the older driver at higher risk for collisions on acceleration and deceleration lanes. This is particularly problematic when traffic volume is high.
- To allow the older driver the greatest advantage for successfully negotiating entrance onto a highway, it is advisable that acceleration lane lengths be increased and that a parallel design for entrance ramps be used to allow enough time for gap search and decision-making processes.
- For exit ramps it is advisable to locate the ramp exits downstream from sight-restricting vertical or horizontal curvature of the main road.

Traffic Control Devices for Restricted or Prohibited Movements on Freeways, Expressways, and Ramps

- Age-related diminished capabilities (particularly selective attention, divided attention, visual acuity, and contrast sensitivity) contribute to wrong-way movements on highways just as they do on other roadways.

- Preventive measures to reduce the frequency of wrong-way movements by older drivers include modification of ramp and roadway design, signing and pavement markers, and use of warning and detection devices and vehicle arresting systems.
- For example, overhead land control signal indicators for prohibited movements (red X) provide conspicuous warning. Guide sign panels marking FREEWAY ENTRANCE provide positive guidance.
- Additionally, median separators with retroreflective markings reduce the change of crossover in areas where entrance and exit ramps are adjacent to each other.

Fixed Lighting

- The effects of aging on the visual system compound the effects of darkness and increase the risk of collision for older drivers, particularly around interchange areas.
- Most notably the declines in visual acuity, contrast sensitivity, glare recovery, and peripheral vision make night driving more difficult for older drivers.
- Increased illumination at interchanges significantly reduces vehicle crashes. Complete interchange lighting is preferred but may not always be feasible. Where complete interchange lighting is not feasible, a partial interchange lighting system may be used.

Roadway Curvature and Passing Zones

Pavement Markings

- Pavement markings and delineation devices provide information about road alignment.
- Under daylight conditions, the markings and delineations should have a high enough effective luminance contrast to the roadway surface to be easily distinguished by older drivers who may have diminished contrast sensitivity.

- During nighttime driving, the use of thick, slightly raised, retroreflective stripes is recommended, as they reflect more light back to the driver under both dry and wet pavement conditions.
- Raised pavement markers applied along the centerline are recommended for sharper curves. Additionally, the use of chevron alignment signs and roadside post-mounted delineation devices provide more information about road curvature.
- For the older driver with lane-keeping difficulties and diminished motor abilities, these pavement markings and delineations can provide needed guidance.

Advanced Signing for Sight-Restricted Locations

- Older drivers have often developed strong expectations about where and when they will encounter road hazards. With well-established expectations and slower reaction time to unexpected information, the older driver often is slower to override an initially incorrect response with a correct response to the hazard.
- When paired with physical changes, the older driver may have diminished ability to execute rapid vehicle control when an emergency maneuver is required.
- Signing that forewarns drivers of potential upcoming hazards can decrease the risk of collision. For example, advanced warning signals paired with yellow placards with PREPARE TO STOP in black clue drivers into an upcoming signalized intersection that may be obscured by vertical or horizontal curvature of the road.

Passing Zones and Passing/Overtaking Lanes on Two-Way Highways

- The most conservative minimum required passing sight distance should be used to accommodate age-related difficulties in judging gaps, longer decision-making time, and protracted reaction time exhibited by older drivers.
- Retroreflective centerline pavement markings supplemented with yellow NO PASSING ZONE

pennants at the beginning of no-passing zones are recommended. When passing/overtaking lanes (in each direction) are included in two-way highway design, they should be placed at sufficiently long intervals to avoid mid-lane collisions.

Construction Zones

Lane Closure/Lane Transition Practices

- Advanced warning of lane closure, changes in direction of the lateral shift in the travel path, or lane drop must be provided in sufficient time for drivers to make timely decisions, as older adults benefit from longer exposure to stimuli.
- Advanced warning is important for older drivers who require increased time to prepare and initiate a safe merging maneuver rather than an erratic vehicle movement.
- For a work zone on high-speed roadways and divided highways, a supplemental, portable changeable message sign providing displaying a one-phrase message (such as LEFT LANE CLOSED) should be located upstream of the lane closure. At the taper for each lane closure, a flashing-arrow panel indicating lane closure is recommended.
- Abbreviations have the potential to be misunderstood and should be avoided.
- Redundant static signing with high retroreflectance is recommended throughout the entire time period of the lane closure.
- Driving speeds should be reduced in work zones, and channelization (e.g., barriers in transition zones, positive separation) between opposing two-lane traffic on all roadways except residential should be used.
- To accommodate the needs of older drivers, channelizing devices include traffic cones with bands of retroreflective material for nighttime operation, tubular markers with a band of retroreflective material, striped vertical panels, chevron panels, and drums with high-brightness sheeting for orange and white retroreflective stripes.

Portable, Changeable Message Signs

- Changeable message signs are effective only if they are conspicuous, legible, and placed where there is least likelihood of being blocked from a motorist's view. The exposure time, or available viewing time, also determines whether the message is acquired by the driver.
- The needs of the older driver should dictate character and letter legibility, legibility distance, and placement. Character and message legibility of changeable message signs should reflect the same considerations as for static signs (i.e., contrast, luminance, color and contrast orientation, font, letter height, letter width, case, stroke width).

Highway–Rail Grade Crossings

- Older drivers with decreased contrast sensitivity and the need for increasing levels of light for night-driving tasks benefit from increasing the detectability and conspicuity of railroad crossing signing and added illumination to passive crossings.
- Detectability and conspicuity can be increased by use of crossbuck posts with white high-brightness retroreflective sheeting, advanced retroreflective pavement markings, post-mounted delineators with high-performance retroreflective sheeting, and the addition of luminaries.

Pedestrians and Age-Related Changes

- Age-related changes that may make it more difficult for older adults to navigate intersections include decreased contrast sensitivity and visual acuity, decreased peripheral vision and "useful field of view," decreased ability to judge safe gaps in traffic, and slowed walking speed.
- Age-related decline in physical strength, joint flexibility, agility, balance, coordination, and endurance may contribute to slower walking speeds and difficulty negotiating curbs.

- Other behaviors of older pedestrians include a greater likelihood to delay before crossing, spending more time at the curb, taking longer to cross the road, and making more head movements before and during crossing.

Crash Types

Crash types that predominantly involve older pedestrians include
- Vehicle turn/merge
- Intersection dash, when a pedestrian appears suddenly in the street in front of an oncoming vehicle at an intersection
- Bus stop–related, in which a pedestrian steps out in front of a stopped bus and is struck by a vehicle moving in the same direction as the bus
- Multiple threats in which one or more vehicles are stopped in a through lane, the pedestrian walks in front of the stopped vehicle and into the path of a vehicle driving in the adjacent lane going in the same direction as the stopped cars.

Possible Prevention Measures

Measures that have been shown to have promise in improving the safety of older pedestrians include
- Use of regulatory signs, such as YIELD TO PEDESTRIANS WHEN TURNING. In some studies, these signs have been effective in reducing the conflicts between turning vehicles that could potentially lead to crashes.
- Exclusive timing or leading pedestrian interval that uses traffic signals to stop motor vehicle traffic in all directions simultaneously for a phase each cycle when pedestrians are allowed to cross the street. Exclusive timing is intended to eliminate turning traffic or other movements that conflict with pedestrians crossing the street.

■ ■ ■

Appendix E.
Historical Perspective on the Role of Occupational Therapy and Driving and Community Mobility

The invention of the mass-produced, power-driven vehicle by Henry Ford in the 1900s began to expand the mobility of people outside their own communities. Although one of the first pieces of adapted driving equipment was introduced in the 1910s (Hyde, 2005), the general public did not have accesss until formal manufacturing of driving adaptive equipment began in the 1950s.

Before the 1970s, people with disabilities had few options for driver education other than through the school systems or commercial driving schools. In the early 1970s, a group of professional driver educators in the school systems who were concerned about this problem started meeting yearly at the annual conference of the American Driver and Traffic Safety Education Association.

Carmella Strano, an occupational therapist from the driving program at Moss Rehabilitation Center in Philadelphia; Dorothy Beard, an occupational therapy assistant from the driving program at the Texas Institute for Rehabilitation and Research in Houston; and Dave Semlow, a kinesotherapist at the Veterans Affairs hospital in Detroit, joined the group of driver educators as they began to address the driving needs of people with various disabilities in their respective rehabilitation centers. In 1977, they decided to meet more formally once a year to discuss their driver evaluation and education work with people with disabilities, and they established the Association of Driver Educators for the Disabled. Today, the organi-zation is called the *Association for Driver Rehabilitation Specialists,* although it has retained its former acronym, *ADED.*

Occupational therapists were instrumental in the growth and development of ADED as a recognized professional organization. In 1987, Susan Pierce was the first woman and the first occupational therapist elected president of the association. Occupational therapists also had a major influence in the development of the ADED certification examination and credentialing program through which one can become a certified driver rehabilitation specialist. At present, there are approximately 300 members of ADED, and about 70% identify themselves as occupational therapists and occupational therapy assistants.

In 1990, occupational therapist Linda Hunt began presenting at the Transportation Research Board meetings regarding her research on driving and dementia. She was awarded grants from NHTSA to evaluate performance of healthy older drivers and those with dementia. Occupational therapist Anne Morris joined Hunt to expand the awareness of driv-ing and community mobility to occupational thera-pists promoting AOTA's partnership with the Trans-portation Research Board.

As the demographics of the U.S. population change in the 21st century, the practice of occupa-tional therapy will have to change to address older adults' community mobility needs. AOTA is working with several health care organizations and government agencies that have recognized the threats and opportunities presented by the aging of the population.

The American Medical Association (AMA) and NHTSA have recognized occupational therapy as a leader in addressing safe mobility for older adults, and AOTA is responding: "AOTA has been working with the medical community to recognize that occupational therapists have the skill set to work with physicians to address the needs of older patients who have questionable driving ability" (NHTSA, 2004, p. 16).

In addition, an increased role for occupational therapy has become a key component of the U.S. Department of Transportation's overall goal of safe mobility for life (Brachtesende, 2003). According to Essie Wagner, a senior analyst with NHTSA, "Safe driving and community mobility are huge societal goals, and occupational therapy is one of the key professions to meet them" (quoted in Green, 2004, p. 44).

The growing recognition of occupational therapy by NHTSA and its working partners, such as AARP and the AMA, places great demand on the profession to develop a plan to meet NHTSA's primary goal of extending "the period of safe driving as well as the development of alternative transportation for those who cannot continue to drive" (NHTSA, 2004, p. 14).

AOTA's Older Driver Initiative is an important element of that plan. Through outreach, advocacy, and federal grants, AOTA's Older Driver Initiative is "positioning the Association and occupational therapy practitioners as leaders in addressing a growing social and public health challenge" (Peterson & Somers, 2003, p. 23).

In 2000, AOTA identified older driver safety as an emerging practice area in its strategic plan. Joining efforts with NHTSA, AOTA held a consensus conference in December 2002 that resulted in recommenda-

tions for increasing occupational therapy's capacity to meet the needs of older drivers. The first task of the initiative was to gather a panel of experts in driving to guide and consult with AOTA as the tasks associated with this project progressed. The expert panel, which met for the first time October 2003, guides the work of the AOTA Older Driver Initiative according to three overall goals:

1. Increase the capacity of occupational therapists to meet the growing needs of older drivers
2. Produce educational and toolkit materials according to the consensus conference recommendations
3. More clearly define occupational therapy's role with older drivers across all practice settings.

The expert panel has participated in strategic planning on behalf of AOTA. The panel defined roles and responsibilities for occupational therapists and occupational therapy assistants in this emerging practice area, and several members have participated in the development of an official AOTA statement on driving and community mobility in collaboration with the Commission on Practice (AOTA, 2005b).

As the practice area becomes more defined, AOTA has developed several mechanisms to support professional growth and continuing competency in driving rehabilitation. These mechanisms include continuing education opportunities, such as an online course, regional workshops, and an annual community mobility symposium. AOTA also has built an older driver microsite to support practitioners, other health care providers, and consumers seeking to advance their knowledge or gather resources. One avenue for obtaining formal recognition as a specialist in driving and community mobility is through AOTA's Driving and Community Specialty Certification (see www.aota.org/certification).

■ ■ ■

Appendix F.
Glossary of Terms Related to Driving and Community Mobility

assistive technology: Any item, piece or equipment, or product system, whether acquired commercially, off the shelf, modified or customized, that is used to increase, maintain, or improve the driving or community mobility capabilities or individuals with disabilities (Assistive Technology Act, 1998).

certified driver rehabilitation specialist: An individual who meets the educational and experiential requirements and successfully completes the certification examination provided by the Association of Driver Rehabilitation Specialists (ADED, 2004).

clinical assessment: The administration of specific tools or instruments used during the first phase of the evaluation process for driving or community mobility. These may include an occupational profile and measures of performance skills, performance patterns, contexts, activity demands, and client factors (AOTA, 2002, 2005a).

community mobility: "Moving [the] self in the community and using private or public transportation, such as driving or accessing buses, taxi cabs, or other public transportation systems" (AOTA, 2002, p. 620).

compromised driving and community mobility: Functional deficits in the performance of driving and community mobility tasks.

driver educator: A professional with a college degree in education with specialized study in driver education.

driver education: A process facilitated by a professional in a classroom and in-vehicle setting whereby a person learns the knowledge, attitude, and skills to be a safe driver.

driver rehabilitation specialist: A specialist who "plans, develops, coordinates, and implements driver rehabilitation services for individuals with disabilities" (ADED, 2004).

driver rehabilitation therapist: An allied health professional with specialized training, experience, and credentials in driver rehabilitation services, including evaluating and training people with disabilities in driving or safe transportation (Pierce, 2002).

driver safety: Operation of a motorized vehicle, with or without adaptive equipment, to travel in a safe manner in coordination with other drivers on public roadways to a desired destination.

driving and community mobility discharge plan: A comprehensive plan that incorporates counseling and mobility management for compromised driving and community mobility that establishes a network of transportation alternatives and identifies of community resources and services.

driving or community mobility evaluation: The entire process of obtaining and interpreting data necessary for intervention related to driving and community mobility. This includes planning for and documenting the evaluation process and results (AOTA, 2005a).

driving instructor: As required by many states, an individual with a high school degree and a clear legal and driving record who has completed a driver education training program and has been licensed as a driving instructor by the state motor vehicle administration.

Federal Motor Vehicle Safety Standards: The NHTSA has a legislative mandate under Title 49 of the U.S. Code, Chapter 301, Motor Vehicle Safety, to issue Federal Motor Vehicle Safety Standards and Regulations to which manufacturers of motor vehicle and equipment items must conform and certify compliance. These federal safety standards are regulations written in terms of minimum safety performance requirements for motor vehicles or items of motor vehicle equipment. The requirements are specified in such a manner "that the public is protected against unreasonable risk of crashes occurring as a result of the design, construction, or performance of motor vehicles and is also protected against unreasonable risk of death or injury in the event crashes do occur" (Federal Motor Vehicle Safety Standards and Regulations, 2004).

instructor safety equipment: Equipment in a driver rehabilitation vehicle used to ensure safety by maximizing visibility and allowing dual vehicle control. This equipment may include an instructor mirror, instructor brake, eye check mirror, and shutoff switches.

in-vehicle or community mobility assessment: The administration of a test of performance skills as it specifically relates to operating a motor vehicle or accessing community mobility conducted in the naturalistic context.

National Mobility Equipment Dealers Standards: A nonprofit trade association of mobility equipment dealers, driver rehabilitation specialists, and other professionals dedicated to broadening the opportunities for people with disabilities to drive or be transported in vehicles modified with mobility equipment. All members work together to improve transportation options of people with disabilities (National Mobility Equipment Dealers Association, 2006).

naturalistic context: The environment and conditions in which driving and community mobility actually occur.

operational demands of driving: Basic control of a motorized vehicle, such as steering, acceleration, and braking functions (Michon, 1985).

paratransit: A form of transportation service that is more flexible and personalized than conventional, fixed-route, or fixed-schedule services. Service is adjusted to individual needs. Examples of paratransit service includes taxis, a jitney, dial-a-ride, vanpool, and subscription services (see http://www.semcog.org/TranPlan/TIPonline/TIPglossary.htm).

referral network: A system of health care providers, law enforcement, court system, social services agencies, state agencies, and related others who collaborate in support of driving and community mobility services.

strategic demands of driving: The highest level of the three demands of driving; involves judgment, planning, and foresight, such as choosing to reschedule a trip because of a snowstorm (Michon, 1985).

tactical demands of driving: Ongoing decisions made while interacting with traffic during driving, such as time and space judgment of a safe gap in traffic in which to execute a left turn (Michon, 1985).

transportation alternatives: Having a choice of more than one means of moving oneself about in the community.

transportation modes: The various means of traveling in the community, including walking and the use of motor and nonmotorized vehicles.

vehicle safety features: Technologies in the automobile designed for occupant protection, including but not limited to, seat belts, airbags, padded dashboards.

■ ■ ■

Appendix G.
Selected *CPT*™ Coding for Occupational Therapy Evaluations and Interventions

The following chart can guide making clinically appropriate decisions in selecting the most relevant *CPT*™ code to describe occupation therapy evaluation and intervention. Occupational therapy practitioners should use the most appropriate code from the current *CPT* based on specific services provided, individual patient goals, payer policy, and common usage.

Examples of Occupational Therapy Evaluation and Intervention	Suggested *CPT*™ Code(s)
• Provide instruction and training in compensatory techniques for performing driving or using community transportation services. • Assist client to incorporate energy conservation techniques to facilitate efficient use of transportation services. • Provide training in use of assistive technology to operate vehicle controls to assure safe, independent driving within the community.	97535—Self-care/home management training (e.g., activities of daily living [ADL] and compensatory training, meal preparation, safety procedures, instructions in use of assistive technology devices/adaptive equipment), direct (one-on-one) contact by the provider, each 15 minutes.
• Assess patient requirements for specialized mobility equipment, such as powered scooters, to enable mobility within the community. • Provide recommendations for wheelchair management and storage in or on the vehicle while driving. • Provide training in wheelchair management and propulsion throughout the community and while using transportation services.	97542—Wheelchair management (e.g., assessment, fitting, training), each 15 minutes.

• Evaluate/assess changes in such areas as
  – Visual skills necessary to see the driving environment or read a transportation schedule.
  – Cognitive-processing abilities for planning and negotiation of busy roadways or transportation systems.
  – Motor performance skills necessary for operation of vehicle controls, mobility within and around transportation vehicles, and adequate balance for safety.
	97003—Occupational therapy evaluation.
	97004—Occupational therapy reevaluation.
	97750—Physical performance test or measurement (e.g., musculoskeletal, functional capacity), with written report, each 15 minutes.

• Provide functional exercises to increase range of motion, strength, and mobility to enable full operation of vehicle controls or accessibility/use of transportation services.	97110—Therapeutic procedure, one or more areas, each 15 minutes. Therapeutic exercises to develop strength and endurance, range of motion, and flexibility.

(continued)

Examples of Occupational Therapy Evaluation and Intervention	Suggested *CPT* Code(s)
• Design graded tasks to increase coordination, balance, and sensory awareness to operate and travel in vehicles.	97112—Therapeutic procedure, one or more areas, each 15 minutes. Neuromuscular reeducation of movement, balance, coordination, kinesthetic sense, posture, and/or proprioception for sitting and/or standing activities.
• Train in use of memory exercises to enhance the ability to remember travel routes, sequencing of steps for complex driving maneuvers, or transportation exchanges. • Develop strategies to improve awareness of the community mobility environment to avoid hazards and preserve the safety of the client, passengers, and other roadway users.	97532—Development of cognitive skills to improve attention, memory, problem solving (includes compensatory training), direct (one-on-one) patient contact by the provider, each 15 minutes.
• Provide occupation-based activities to increase ability to perform driving and community mobility tasks such as route planning and map reading.	97530—Therapeutic activities, direct (one-on-one) patient contact by the provider (use of dynamic activities to improve functional performance), each 15 minutes.
• Teach safe driving techniques on the continuum of roadway complexities and conditions, including residential roads, moderately traveled roads, highways, parking lot entrances and exits, inclement weather, and high traffic. • Provide community mobility activities involving access to community resources such as negotiating a drive-up ATM, traveling through and parking in a busy shopping plaza, refueling an automobile at a gas station, and finding the way to frequently visited destinations.	92537—Community/work reintegration training (e.g., shopping, transportation, money management, avocational activities and/or work environment/modification analysis, work task analysis, use of assistive technology device/adaptive equipment), direct one-on-one contact by the provider, each 15 minutes.
• Assess the utility of an orthotic or prosthetic while operating a motor vehicle or using transportation services. • Recommend changes to a prosthetic terminal device for compatibility with driving assistive technology. • Recommend a accelerator pedal block to prevent accidental operation with a lower-extremity prosthesis. • Provide exercises to improve effectiveness, efficiency, and safety of community mobility transfers while wearing an orthotic or prosthesis.	97760—Orthotic(s) management and training (including assessment and fitting when not otherwise reported), upper extremity(s), lower extremity(s) and/or trunk, each 15 minutes. 97762—Checkout for orthotic/prosthetic use, established patient, each 15 minutes.
• Provide joint mobilization to the shoulder to increase joint range of motion to move a steering wheel through a full rotation.	97140—Manual therapy techniques (e.g., mobilization/manipulation, manual lymphatic drainage, manual traction), one or more regions, each 15 minutes.
• Assess a client with paraplegia for ability to safely and effectively use assistive technology for operating an automobile or accessing/using transit, including but not limited to computer controlled acceleration/braking equipment, computerized ignition systems, wheelchair lifts, and hand controls.	97755 Assistive technology assessment.

Note. The *CPT* 2006 codes referenced in this chart do not represent all of the possible codes that may be used in occupational therapy evaluation and intervention. Not all payers will reimburse for all codes. Refer to *CPT 2006* for the complete list of available codes.

CPT™ is a trademark of the American Medical Association (AMA). *CPT* 5-digit codes, nomenclature, and other data are copyright © 2005 by the American Medical Association. All rights reserved. Reprinted with permission. No fee schedules, basic units, relative values, or related listings are included in *CPT*. The AMA assumes no liability for the data contained herein.

Codes shown refer to *CPT 2006*. CPT codes are updated annually. New and revised codes become effective January 1. Always refer to annual updated *CPT* publication for most current codes.

References

Allen, C. K. (1996). *Allen cognitive level tests manual.* Colchester, CT: S&S Worldwide.

American Association of Retired Persons. (2003). Beyond 50 2003: Report to the nation on independent living and disability. Washington, DC: Authors.

American Occupational Therapy Association. (1979). Uniform terminology for occupational therapy services. *Occupational Therapy News, 35*(11), 1–8.

American Occupational Therapy Association. (1989). Uniform terminology for occupational therapy (2nd ed.). *American Journal of Occupational Therapy, 43,* 808–815.

American Occupational Therapy Association. (1994). Uniform terminology for occupational therapy (3rd ed.). *American Journal of Occupational Therapy, 43,* 1047–1054.

American Occupational Therapy Association. (1999a). Standards for an accreditededucational program for the occupational therapist. *American Journal of Occupational Therapy, 53,* 573–582.

American Occupational Therapy Association. (1999b). Standards for an accredited educational program for the occupational therapy assistant. *American Journal of Occupational Therapy, 53,* 583–589.

American Occupational Therapy Association. (2002). Occupational therapy practice framework: Domain and process. *American Journal of Occupational Therapy, 56,* 609–639.

American Occupational Therapy Association. (2003). Guidelines for documentation of occupational therapy. *American Journal of Occupational Therapy, 57,* 646–649.

American Occupational Therapy Association. (2004). Guidelines for supervision, roles and responsibilities during the delivery of occupational therapy services. *American Journal of Occupational Therapy, 58,* 663–667.

American Occupational Therapy Association. (2005a). Standards of practice for occupational therapy, *American Journal of Occupational Therapy, 59,* 663–665.

American Occupational Therapy Association. (2005b). Statement: Driving and community mobility. *American Journal of Occupational Therapy, 59,* 666–670.

American Occupational Therapy Association. (2006). Policy 1.44: Categories of occupational therapy personnel. In *Policy manual* (2005 ed.). Bethesda, MD: Author. Retrieved August 2, 2006, from http://www.aota.org/members/area6/docs/pm_1205.pdf.

Americans with Disabilities Act of 1990, P.L. 101–336, 104 Stat. 328 (1991).

Arbesman M., Campbell, R. M., & Rhynders, P. A. (2001). The role of occupational therapy in injury prevention. *Israel Journal of Occupational Therapy, 10*(4), 97–108.

Assistive Technology Act of 1998, P.L. 105–394.

Association for Driver Rehabilitation Specialists. (2004). *Best practices for delivery of driver rehabilitation services.* Ruston, LA: Author. (www.aded.org)

Avorn, J. (1995). Medication use and the elderly: Current status and opportunities. *Health Affairs, 14,* 276–286.

Baron, K., Kielhofner, G., Lyenger, A., Goldhammer, V., & Wolenski, J. (2006). *Occupational Self Assessment* (OSA, Version 2.2). Chicago: University of Illinois at Chicago. MOHO Clearinghouse.

Beard, J. G., & Ragheb, M. G. (1980). The Leisure Satisfaction Questionnaire. *Journal of Leisure Research, 12*, 20–32.

Berg, J. (1997). Playing the outcomes game. *OT Week, 11*(22), 12–15.

Berkman, L. F., & Tinetti, M. E. (1997). Driving cessation and increased depressive symptoms: Prospective evidence from the New Haven EPESE. *Journal of the American Geriatrics Society, 45*, 202–206.

Blessed, G., Tomlinson, B. E., & Roth, M. (1968). The association between quantitative measures of dementia and of senile change in the cerebral gray matter of elderly subjects. *British Journal of psychiatry, 114*, 797–811.

Brachtesende, A. (2003). Ready to go? Community mobility issues of older adults. *OT Practice, 8*(18), 14–25.

Brink, T. L., Yesavaage, J. A., Lum, O., Heersema, P., Adey, M. B., & Rose, T. L. (1982). Screening tests for geriatric depression. *Clinical Gerontologist, 1*, 37–44.

Burns, N. R., Nettlebeck, T., White, M., & Wilson, J. (1999). Effects of car window tinting on visual performance: A comparison of elderly and young drivers. *Ergonomics, 42*, 428–443.

Carlson, P. J. (2001). *Evaluation of Clearview alphabet with microprismatic retroreflective sheetings* (FHWA Report # FHWA/TX-02/4049-1). Springfield, VA: National Technical Information Service.

Carmeli, E., Coleman, R., Omar, H. L., & Brown-Cross, D. (2000). Do we allow elderly pedestrians sufficient time to cross the street in safety? *Journal of Aging and Physical Activity, 8*, 51–58.

Carr, D. B., Labarge, E., Dunnigan, K., & Storandt, M. (1998). Differentiating drivers with dementia of the Alzheimer's type from healthy older persons with a traffic sign naming test. *Journal of Gerontology: A Biological Science Medical Science, 53*, M135–M139.

Center for Functional Assessment Research at the State University of New York at Buffalo. (1993). *Functional Independence Measure* (4th ed.). Buffalo, NY: Data Management Service of the Uniform Data System for Medical Rehabilitation.

Center for Injury Prevention Policy and Practice. (2002). *Traffic safety among older adults: recommendations for California.* San Diego: San Diego State University.

Christoffel, T., & Gallagher, S. C. (1999). *Injury prevention and public health.* Gaithersburg, MD: Aspen.

Chrysler, S. T., Carlson, P. J., & Hawkins, H. G. (2002). *Nighttime legibility of ground-mounted signs as a function of font, color, and retroreflective sheeting type* (FHWA Report #FHWA/TX-03/1796-2). Springfield, VA: National Technical Information Service.

Clay, O.J., Wadley, V.G., Edwards, J.D., Roth, D.L., Roenker, D.L., & Ball, K.K. (2005). Cumulative meta-analysis of the relationship between useful field of view and driving performance in older adults: Current and future implications. *Optometry and Vision Science, 82*, 724–731.

Colarusso, R. P., & Hammill, D. D. (2003). *Motor-Free Visual Perception Test* (MVPT–3, 3rd ed.). Novato, CA: Academic Therapy Publications.

Darwish, D., & Hagin, R. A. (1995). Clock Drawing Test: Establishing normative standards foruse in psychosocial assessment. *Learning Disabilities: A Multidisciplinary Journal, 6*, 31–39.

Dubinsky, R. M., Stein, A. C., & Lyons, K. (2000). Practice parameter: Risk of driving and Alzheimer's disease (an evidence-based review): Report of the Quality Standards Subcommittee of the American Academy of Neurology. *Neurology, 54*, 2205–2211.

Dunn, W., Brown, C., & McGuigan, A. (1994). The ecology of human performance: A framework for considering the effect of context. *American Journal of Occupational Therapy, 48*, 595–607.

Dunn, W., McClain, L. H., Brown, C., & Youngstrom, M. J. (1998). The ecology of human performance. In M. E. Neistadt & E. B. Crepeau (Eds.), *Willard and Spackman's occupational therapy* (9th ed., pp. 525–535). Philadelphia: Lippincott Williams & Wilkins.

Fancher, P., Ervin, R., Sayer, J., Hagan, M., Bogard, S., Bareket, Z., et al. (1998). *Intelligent Cruise Control Field Operational Test* (Final Report, Report No. UMTRI-98-17). Ann Arbor: University of Michigan, Transportation Research Institute.

Federal Interagency Forum of Aging-Related Statistics. (2000). *Older Americans 2000: Key indicators of well-being detailed many other statistical indicators of the health and economic needs of future older Americans.* Retrieved from www.agingstats.gov/chartbook2000/default.htm.

Fischer, A. G. (1995). *Assessment of Motor and Process Skills.* Fort Collins, CO: Three Star Press.

Fisher, A., & Kielhofner, G. (1995). Skill in occupational performance. In G. Kielhofner (Ed.), *A model of human occupation: Theory and application* (pp. 113–128). Philadelphia: Lippincott Williams & Wilkins.

Florey, L. & Michelman, S. M. (1982). The Occupational Role History: A screening tool for psychiatric occupational therapy. *American Journal of Occupational Therapy, 36,* 301–308.

Folstein, M. F., Folstein, S. E., & McHugh, P. R. (1975). Mini-Mental State: A practical method for grading the state of patients for the clinician. *Journal of Psychiatric Research, 12,* 189–198.

Freedman, M., Zador, P., & Staplin, L. (1993). Effects of reduced transmittance film on automobile rear window visibility. *Human Factors, 35,* 535–550.

Freund, K. (2002). *Pilot testing innovative payment operations for independent transportation for the elderly* (Final Report for Transit-IDEA Project 18). Washington, DC: Transportation Research Board.

Gardner, M. F. (1993). *Test of Visual–Perceptual Skills (Non-Motor): Upper Level.* Burlingame, CA: Psychological and Educational Publications.

Gartman, D. (2004). Three ages of the automobile: The cultural logics of the car. *Theory, Culture, and Society, 21*(4/5), 169–195.

Grabowski, D. C., Campbell, C. M., & Morrisey, M. A. (2004). Elderly licensure laws and motor vehicle fatalities. *Journal of the American Medical Association, 291,* 2840–2846.

Green, N. (2204). It takes a village. *OT Practice, 9*(7), 44.

Hakamies-Blomqvist, L., Johansson, K., & Lundburg, C. (1996). Medical screening of older drivers as a traffic safety measure: A comparative Finnish–Swedish evaluation study. *Journal of the American Geriatrics Society, 44,* 650–653.

Havighurst, R. J. (1961). Successful aging. *The Gerontologist, 1,* 8–13.

Hing, J. Y., Stamatiadis, N., & Autman-Hall, L. (2003). Evaluating the impact of passengers on the safety of older drivers. *Journal of Safety Research, 34,* 343–351.

Ho, G., Scialfa, C. T., Caird, J. K., & Graw, T. (2001). Visual search for traffic signs: The effects of clutter, luminance, and aging. *Human Factors, 43,* 194–207.

Hooper, H. E. (1958). *Hooper Visual Organization Test.* Los Angeles: Western Psychological Services.

Hopkins, H. L., & Smith, H. D. (1985). *Willard and Spackman's occupational therapy.* Philadelphia: Lippincott.

Hunt, L. (2001). *National Traffic Highway Administration Report (NHTSA).* Retrieved May 25, 2005, from http://dms.dot.gov/search/document.cfm?documentid=138293&docketid=3588.

Hunt, L. (2005, December). *Is there an answer to the dementia and driving problem?* Paper presented at the 2nd Annual Community Mobility Symposium, Orlando, FL.

Hunt, L. A., Morris, J. C., Edwards, D. F., & Wilson, B. (1993). Driving performance in persons with mild senile dementia of the Alzheimer's type. *Journal of the American Geriatrics Society, 41,* 747–753.

Hunt, L. A., Murphy, C. F., Carr, D., Duchek, J. M., Buckles, V., & Morris, J. C. (1997a). Environmental cueing may affect performance on a road test for drivers with dementia of the Alzheimer type. *Alzheimer Disease and Associated Disorders, 11* (Suppl. 1).

Hunt, L. A., Murphy, C. F., Carr, D., Duchek, J. M., Buckles, V., & Morris, J. C. (1997b). Reliability of the Washington University road test. *Archives of Neurology, 54,* 707–712.

Hyde, C. L. (2005). History of the automobile. In J. Pellerito (Ed.), *Driver rehabilitation and community mobility—Principles and practice* (pp. 23–33). St. Louis, MO: Elsevier Mosby.

Karagiozis, H., Gray, S., Sacco, J., Shapiro, M., & Kawas, C. (1998). Direct assessment of adult functional abilities (DAFA): A comparison to an indirect measure of instrumental activities of daily living. *The Gerontologist, 38,* 113–121.

Katzman, R., Brown, T., Fuld, P., Peck, A., Schechter, R., & Schimmel, H. (1983). Validation of a short-orientation–memory-concentration test of cognitive impairment. *American Journal Psychiatry, 140,* 734–739.

Kautzmann, L. N. (1984). Identifying leisure interests: A self-assessment approach for adults with arthritis. *Occupational Therapy in Health Care, 1*(2), 45–52.

Kielhofner, G., Henry, A. D., & Whalens, D. (1989). *Occupational Performance History Interview.* Bethesda, MD: American Occupational Therapy Association.

Kiernan, R. J., Mueller, J., Langston, J. W., & Van Dyke, C. (1987). The Neurobehavioral Cognitive Status Examination: A brief but differentiated approach to cognitive assessment. *Annals of Internal Medicine, 107,* 481–485.

Klavora, P., Gaskovski, P., Martin, K., Forsyth, R. D., Heslegrave, R. J., Young, M., et al. (1995). The effects of dynavision rehabilitation on behind-the-wheel driving ability and selected psychomotor abilities of persons after stroke. *American Journal of Occupational Therapy, 49,* 534–542.

Kline, D. W., Buck, K., Sell, Y., Bolan, T. L., & Dewar, R. E. (1999). Older observers' tolerance of optical blur: Age differences in the identification of defocused text signs. *Human Factors, 48,* 356–364.

Kloseck, M., & Crilly, R. G. (1987). *Leisure Competency Measure: Adult version.* London, Ontario: Data System.

Korner-Bitensky, N. A., Sofer, S., Gelinas., I., & Mazer, B. L. (1998). Brief or New: Evaluating driving in persons with stroke: A survey of occupational therapy practices. *American Journal of Occupational Therapy, 52,* 916–919.

LaMotte, J., Ridder III, W., Yeung, K., & De Land, P. (2000). Effect of aftermarket automobile window tinting films on driver vision. *Human Factors, 42,* 327–336.

Laux, L. F. (1991). *Locating vehicle controls and displays: Effects of expectancy and age.* Washington, DC: AAA Foundation for Traffic Safety.

Law, M. (Ed.). (2002). *Evidence-based rehabilitation: A guide to practice.* Thorofare, NJ: Slack.

Law, M., Baptiste, S., Carswell, A., McColl, M., Polatajko, H., & Pollock, (1998). *Canadian Occupational Performance Measure manual* (3rd ed.). Ottawa, Ontario: CAOT Publications.

Law, M., & Baum, C. (1998). Evidence-based occupational therapy. *Canadian Journal of Occupational Therapy, 65,* 131–135.

Li, G., Braver, E. R., & Chen, L. H. (2003). Fragility versus excessive crash involvement as determinants of high death rates per vehicle-mile of travel among older drivers. *Accident Analysis and Prevention, 35,* 227–235.

Llaneras, R. E., Swezey, R. W., Brock, J. F., Rogers, W. C., & Van Cott, H. P. (1998). Enhancing the safe driving performance of older commercial vehicle drivers. *International Journal of Industrial Ergonomics, 22,* 217–245.

Lowenstein, D. A., Amigo, E., Duara, R., Gutterman, A., Hurwitz, D., Berkowitz, N. et al. (1989). A new scale for the assessment of functional status in Alzheimer's disease and related disorders. *Journal of Gerontology, 4,* 114–121.

Machurin, R. K., DeBittignies, B. H., & Pirozzolo, F. J. (1991). Structured assessment of independent living skills: Preliminary report of a performance measure of functional abilities in dementia. *Journal of Gerontology Psychological Science, 46,* 58–66.

Mandel, D. R., Jackson, J. M., Zemke, R., Nelson, L., & Clark, F. A. (Eds.). (1999). *Lifestyle redesign: Implementing the Well Elderly Program.* Bethesda, MD: American Occupational Therapy Association.

Marottoli, R. A., Mendes de Leon, C. F., Glass, T. A., Williams, C. S.,.Berkman, L. F., et al. (1997). Driving cessation and increased depressive symptoms: Prospective evidence from the New Haven EPESE. *Journal of the American Geriatrics Society, 45,* 202–206.

Marshall, S. C., Spasoff, R., Nair, R., & Walraven, C. (2002). Restricted driver licensing for medical impairments: Does it work? *Canadian Medical Association Journal, 167,* 747–751.

Mazer, B. L., Sofer, S., Korner-Bitensky, N., Gelinas, I., Hanley, J., & Wood-Dauphinee, S. (2003). Effectiveness of a visual attention retraining program on the driving performance of clients with stroke. *Archives of Physical Medicine Rehabilitation, 84,* 541–550.

Meyers, J. E., & Meyers, K. R. (1995). *Rey Complex Figure Test and Recognition Trial.* Lutz, FL: Psychological Assessment Resources.

Michon, J. A. (1985). A critical view of driver behavior models: What do we know, what should we do? In L. Evans & R. C. Schwing (Eds.), *Human behavior and traffic safety* (pp. 485–520). New York: Plenum Press.

Minkelm, J. L. (1995, September). *Assistive technology and outcome measurement: Where do we begin?* Symposium conducted at the Canadian Seating and Mobility Conference, Toronto, Ontario.

Morris, J. C. (1993). The Clinical Dementia Rating (CDR): Current version and scoring rules. *Neurology, 43,* 2412–2414.

Morris, J. C. (1997). Clinical Dementia Rating: A reliable and valid diagnostic and staging measure for dementia of the Alzheimer type. *International Psychogeriatrics, 9*(Suppl. 1), 173–178.

Mosey, A. C. (1996). *Applied scientific inquiry in the health professions: An epistemological orientation* (2nd ed.). Bethesda, MD: American Occupational Therapy Association.

Moyers, P. A. (1999). The guide to occupational therapy practice. *American Journal of Occupational Therapy, 53*(3).

National Center for Health Statistics (2004). *NCHS Deaths: Inquiries 2001.* (National Vital Statistics Reports, 52[21]). Retrieved from www.cdc.gov/nchs/fastats/acc-inj.htm.

National Highway Traffic Safety Administration. (2003). *Traffic safety facts 2002: Older population.* Available from http://www-nrd.nhtsa.dot.gov/pdf/nrd-30/NCSA/TSF2002/2002oldfacts.pdf.

National Highway Traffic Safety Administration. (2004). Driver rehabilitation: A growing niche. *OT Practice, 9*(9), 13–18.

National Mobility Equipment Dealers Association. (2006). *National Mobility Equipment Dealers Association.* Retrieved April 13, 2006, from http://www.nmeda.org

Norbeck, J. S., Lindsey, A. M., & Carrieri, V. L. (1981). The development of an instrument to measure social support. *Nursing Research, 32*(1), 4–9.

Oakley, F., Kielhofner, G., Barris, R., & Reichler, R. K. (1986). The Role Checklist: Development and empirical assessment of reliability. *Occupational Therapy Journal of Research, 6,* 157–169.

Ostrow, A. C., Shafron, P., & McPherson, K. (1992). The effects of a joint range-of-motion physical fitness training program on the automatic driving skills of older adults. *Journal of Safety Research, 23,* 207–219.

Ott, B. R., Anthony, D., Papandonatos, G. D., D'Abreu, A., Burock, J., Curtin, A., et al. (2005). Clinician assessment of the driving competence of patients with dementia. *Journal of the American Geriatrics Society, 53,* 829–833.

Owsley, C., Stalvey, B., Wells, J., & Sloane, M. E. (1999). Older drivers and cataract: Driving habits and crash risk. *Journal of Gerontology: Medical Sciences, 54A,* M203–M211.

Parnham, L. D., & Fazio, L. S. (Eds.). (1997). *Play in occupational therapy for children.* St. Louis: Mosby.

Pellerito, J. M., Jr. (2005). *Driver rehabilitation and community mobility: Principles and practice.* Philadelphia: Elsevier Mosby.

Peterson, M. F., & Somers, F. P. (2003). Older driver opportunities. *OT Practice, 8*(21), 23–24.

Phelan, E. A., Anderson, L. A., Lacroix, A. Z., & Larson, E. B. (2004). Older adults' views of "successful aging"—How do they compare with researchers' definitions? *Journal of the American Geriatric Society, 52,* 211–216.

Pierce, S. L. (2002). Driving as an instrumental activity of daily living. In G. Gillen & A. Burkhardt (Eds.), *Stroke: A function-based approach* (2nd ed., pp. 490–498). St. Louis, MO: Moshy.

Pierce, S. L., & Hunt, L. A. (2004). *Driving and community mobility for older adults: Occupational therapy roles* [Online Course]. Bethesda, MD: American Occupational Therapy Association.

Pike, J. (2004). Reducing injuries and fatalities to older drivers: Vehicle concepts. In *Transportation in an aging society: A decase of experience (Technical Papers and Reports From a Conference,* pp. 213–226). Washington, DC: Transportation Reseaerch Board.

Portney, L. G., & Watkins, M. P. (2000). *Foundations of clinical research: Applications to practice* (2nd ed.). Upper Saddle River, NJ: Prentice Hall.

Ragland, D. R., Satariano, W. A., MacLeod, K. E. (2005). Driving cessation and increased depressive symptoms. *Journals of Gerontology: Medical Sciences, 60A,* 399–403.

Reitan, R. M. (1958). Validity of the Trail Making Test as an indication of organic brain damage. *Perceptual and Motor Skills, 8,* 271–276.

Reitan, R. M., & Wolfson, D. 2004. *Comprehensive handbook of psychological assessment, Volume 1. Intellectual and Neuropsychological Assessment,* G. Goldstein & S. Beers, Eds.). Hoboken, NJ: John Wiley & Sons.

Riopel, N., & Kielhofner, G. (1986). *Occupational Questionnaire.* Chicago: University of Illinois at Chicago, MOHO Clearing House.

Roenker, L. L., Cissell, G. M., Ball, K. K., Wadley, V. G., & Edwards, J. D. (2003). Speed-of-processing and driving simulator training result in improved driving performance. *Human Factors, 45,* 218–233.

Rogers, J., & Holm, M. (1994). Assessment of self-care. In B. R. Bonder & M. G. Wagner (Eds.), *Functional performance in older adults* (pp. 181–202). Philadelphia: F. A. Davis.

Rosenbloom, S. (1999, November). *The mobility of the elderly: There's good news and bad news.* Paper presented at the Transportation in an Aging Society: A Decade of Experience, Washington, DC.

Runyan, C. W. (1998). Using the Haddon matrix: Introducing the third dimension. *Injury Prevention, 4,* 302–307.

Sackett, D. L. (1986). Rules of evidence and clinical recommendations on use of antithrombotic agents. *Chest, 89*(Suppl. 2), 2S–3S.

Schold Davis, E. (2003). Defining OT roles in driving. *OT Practice 8*(1), 15–18.

Schumann, J., Flannagan, M. J., Sivak, M., & Traube, E. C. (1997). Daytime veiling glare and driver visual performance: Influence of windshield rake angle and dashboard reflectance. *Journal of Safety Research, 28,* 133–146.

Sheller, M. (2004). Automotive emotions: Feeling the car. *Theory, Culture, and Society, 21,* 221–242.

Shipp, M. D. (1998). Potential human and economic cost-savings attributable to vision testing policies for driver license renewal, 1989–1991. *Optometry and Vision Science, 75,* 103–118.

Smith, A. (1973). *Symbol Digit Modalities Test manual.* Los Angeles: Western Psychological Services.

Staplin, L., Lococo, K., Byington, S., & Harkey, D. (2001). *Highway design handbook for older drivers and pedestrians.* (Pub. No. FHWA-RD-01-103). Washington, DC: U.S. Department of Transportation, Federal Highway Administration.

Stav, W. (2004, May 20). *Assessment of driver–vehicle fit: Part of a comprehensive driving evaluation.* Paper presented at the American Occupational Therapy Association Annual Conference, Minneapolis, MN.

Taylor, B. D., & Tripodes, S. (2001). The effects of driving cessation on the elderly with dementia and their caregivers. *Accident Analysis and Prevention, 33,* 519–528.

Thomson, L. K. (1992). *Kohlman Evaluation of Living Skills* (3rd ed.). Bethesda, MD: American Occupational Therapy Association.

Trenerry, M. R., Crosson, B., DeBoe, J. B., & Leber, W. R. (1989). *Stroop Neuropsychological Screening Test.* Odessa, FL: Psychological Assessment Resources.

Trombly, C. A. (1995). Occupation: purposefulness and meaningfulness as therapeutic mechanisms. *American Journal of Occupational Therapy, 49,* 960–972.

U.S. Department of Transportation. (2003). *Safe mobility for a maturing society: Challenges and opportunities.* Washington, DC: Author.

Urry, J. (2004). The system of automobility. *Theory, Culture, and Society, 21*(4/5), 25–39.

Uttl, B., & Pilkenton-Taylor, C. (2001). Letter cancellation performance across the adult life span. *Clinical Neuropsychology, 15,* 521–530.

Vollrath, M., Meilinger, T., & Kruger, H. (2002). How the presence of passengers influences the risk of a collision with another vehicle. *Accident Analysis and Prevention, 34,* 649–654.

Wang, C. C., Kosinski, C. J., Schwartzberg, J. G., & Shanklin, A. V. (2003). *Physician's guide to assessing and counseling older drivers.* Washington, DC: National Highway Traffic Safety Administration.

Watanabe, S. (1968). Activities configuration social adaptation: "Making it." In American Occupational Therapy Association, Region VI Council on Practice (Ed.), *Evaluation procedures in community health programs: Pere Marquettte State Park, Grafton, IL, May 18–19, 1968.* Rockville, MD: American Occupational Therapy Association.

Wechsler, D. (1997). *Wechsler Adult Intelligence Scale–Revised.* San Antonio, TX: Harcourt Assessment.

Witt, P. A., & Ellis, G. D. (1984). The Leisure Diagnostic Battery: Measuring perceived freedom in leisure. *Society and Leisure, 7,* 109–124.

Wood-Dauphinee, S., Opzoomer, A., Williams, J. L., Marchand, B., & Spitzer, W. O. (1988). Assessment of global function: The Reintegration to Normal Living Index. *Archives of Physical Medicine and Rehabilitation, 69,* 583–590.

World Health Organization. (2001). *International classification of functioning, disability, and health.* Geneva: Author.